The Sentinel Node in Surgical Oncology

Springer

Berlin
Heidelberg
New York
Barcelona
Hong Kong
London
Milan
Paris
Singapore
Tokyo

M.R.S. Keshtgar
W.A. Waddington
S.R. Lakhani
P.J. Ell

The Sentinel Node in Surgical Oncology

With a Foreword by
I. Taylor and M. Baum

With Contributions by
P.C. Barneveld · V. Bongers · I.H.M. Borel Rinkers
A.J. Britten · M.R. Canninga-van Dijk · E. Howard-Jones · G. Kocjan
P.P. van Rijk · W.A. van Vloten

With 363 Illustrations
157 in Full Color

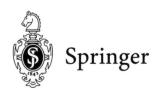

Springer

Mohammad R.S. Keshtgar, BSc, MB, BS, FRCSI, FRGS(Gen)
Clinical Lecturer/Surgical Oncologist
Institute of Nuclear Medicine
Royal Free and University College Medical School
University College London
Mortimer Street, London W1N 8AA, UK

Wendy A. Waddington, BSc, MSc, MIPEM
Principal Nuclear Medicine Physicist
Institute of Nuclear Medicine
Royal Free and University College Medical School
University College London
Mortimer Street, London W1N 8AA, UK

Sunil R. Lakhani, BSc, MB, BS, MD, MRCPath
Senior Lecturer and Consultant
Department of Histopathology
Royal Free and University College Medical School
University College London
Rockefeller Building, University Street, London WC1E 6JJ, UK

Peter J. Ell, MD, PD, MSc, FRCR, FRCP
Professor and Head of Institute of Nuclear Medicine
Royal Free and University College Medical School
University College London
Mortimer Street, London W1N 8AA, UK

ISBN 3-540-65176-4 Springer-Verlag Berlin Heidelberg New York

Library of Congress Cataloging-in-Publication Data

The sentinel node in surgical oncology / [edited by] M.R.S. Keshtgar ... [et al.] ; with contributions by P.C. Barneveld ... [et al.]. p.   cm. Includes bibliographical references and index. ISBN 3-540-65176-4 (alk. paper). 1. Lymphatic metastasis–Radionuclide imaging. I. Keshtgar, M., R. S. (Mohammad R. S.). 1962-   . II. Barneveld. P.C. (Peter C.) [DNLM: 1. Neoplasms–diagnosis. 2. Lymph Nodes–radionuclide imaging. 3. Radiopharma-ceuticals–diagnostic use. 4. Lymphatic Metastasis–radionuclide imaging.   QZ 241 S478 1999] RD598.8.S46   1999. 616.99'407575–dc21. DNLM/DLC for Library of Congress. 98-52045

Cover design: Erich Kirchner, Heidelberg
Typesetting: Fotosatz-Service Köhler GmbH, 97084 Würzburg
Computer to film and binding: Konrad Triltsch, Druck- und Verlagsanstalt GmbH, 97070 Würzburg

SPIN: 10693790   21/3135 - 5 4 3 2 1 0 - Printed on acid-free paper

Foreword

Every so often a concept emerges in the management of solid malignancy that is rapidly incorporated into practice or alters our perception of treatment and accordingly has the potential to influence treatment algorithms significantly. Sentinel lymph node scintigraphy and biopsy represent a classic example. This method was initially introduced for the management of malignant melanoma and rapidly proved to be popular and valuable. It has subsequently been applied to breast cancer and its popularity has spread with almost indecent haste. With increasing experience it is becoming apparent that the technique, whilst of potential value, nevertheless requires fastidious performance if it is to be effective, and it must be assessed carefully. Demonstration of proven efficacy is necessary if it is to be incorporated into general surgical practice. What do we mean by efficacy in this case? Up until about 30 years ago surgical clearance of the axilla was considered essential as a life-saving component of the radical management of primary breast cancer. Since then, however, we have become more modest in our objectives. We now look upon axillary node dissection as primarily a means of controlling the disease locally, whilst at the same time providing valuable prognostic information to make decisions about adjuvant systemic therapy or for counselling the patient in other ways. As breast cancer is being diagnosed at earlier and earlier stages, the positivity of the axilla after radical clearance has fallen to a level of about 30%. This means that up to 70% of patients with primary breast cancer are undergoing unnecessary axillary dissection with its subsequent morbidity for no particular return. At the same time, is adjuvant chemotherapy being recommended to more and more patients with negative axillae, particularly amongst the pre-menopausal group, in spite of a negative lymph node status. Ideally, therefore, we need some procedure that will allow us to avoid unnecessary radical treatment of the negative axilla, whilst allowing us to make borderline decisions about the role of adjuvant systemic therapies amongst patients at the more favourable end of the spectrum of prognosis. It is in this area that the sentinel node biopsy is likely to prove its worth, but not until it has been subjected to a large, pragmatic, randomised controlled trial, comparing unselected axillary node clearance and management dependent on the outcome of the sentinel node biopsy. Such a trial has just been funded by the Medical Research Council in the UK, and it is to be conducted through the UK Co-ordinating Committee for Cancer Research (UKCCCR).

This excellent book reviews all aspects of sentinel lymph node scintigraphy and biopsy. It covers in an admirable fashion practical aspects such as how to choose a probe, which radiopharmaceutical agent to use, how imaging should be performed and, particularly, the surgical techniques involved if optimum results are to be achieved. Undoubtedly, the histology and cytology of the excised sentinel lymph node are of the utmost importance and require expert interpretation. This aspect is covered in detail and the many pitfalls highlighted. The authors have also provided the reader with the benefits of their experience by including excellent illustrative case reports to demonstrate the various practical aspects of the technique. We congratulate the authors on an excellent review of this topic, which could alter our management of patients with common solid malignancies.

I. TAYLOR
M. BAUM

Preface

Medicine is at its best when it can attract a multidisciplinary team to the solution of an important patient-related problem. It can be stated without equivocation that patient selection is amongst the top priorities since only then can appropriate resources be matched to the appropriate management of disease.

This book is the result of such a multidisciplinary effort. A general surgeon with an interest in cancer, a general nuclear medicine physician, a medical physicist and a pathologist have teamed up to bring into focus the present role of lymphoscintigraphy and the detection of the sentinel lymph node in the surgical management of cancer.

The combined expertise is significant. The bridge to span (surgical procedures and the operating theatre environment, radiation detectors and imaging devices and their safe operation, radiopharmaceuticals and their appropriate selection and use, pathological evidence gathering and interpretation and last but certainly not least, effective clinical decision making) is wide, and the subject of this succinct and focussed text.

It is our combined hope that by scanning through the pages of this volume, surgeons, general and nuclear medicine physicians, radiologists and radiation health workers, will all find relevant information that is presented in a concise and hopefully also critical manner.

This volume also represents another example of the power of modern tracer technology in medicine. As more data are gathered in this rapidly expanding field it is already time to consider how we can all improve existing methodologies. Patients will clearly be the main beneficiaries.

M. R. S. KESHTGAR
W. A. WADDINGTON
S. R. LAKHANI
P. J. ELL

Acknowledgements

We wish to acknowledge the contributions by

Peter C. Barneveld, Vivian Bongers, Inne H. M. Borel Rinkers, Allan J. Britton, Marijke R. Canninga-van Dijk, Elliott Howard-Jones, Gabrijella Kocjan, Peter P. van Rijk, Willem A. van Vloten (for addresses see p. XIII).

We wish to acknowledge further:

Prof. I. Taylor, Prof. M. Baum, Miss C. Saunders, from the Academic Division of Surgical Specialities, Royal Free and University College Medical School, Mr. T. Davidson, Consultant Surgeon from the Royal Free Hospital and Dr. M. Spittle, Consultant Oncologist, UCLH Trust Hospitals for the referral of patients,

and

the significant assistance from M. Dashwood (Department of Molecular Pathology and Clinical Biochemistry) and G. Landon, (Department of Histopathology), both from Royal Free and University College Medical School, London, H. Jones (photography, illustration and AV Centre, UCL) and C. Murrain and F. MacSweeney (Institute of Nuclear Medicine, Royal Free and University College Medical School).

Contents

Contributors

PETER C. BARNEVELD, MD
Department of Nuclear Medicine
University Hospital Utrecht
P. O. Box 85500
3508 GA Utrecht
The Netherlands

VIVIAN BONGERS, MD
Department of Nuclear Medicine
University Hospital Utrecht
P.O. Box 85500
3508 GA Utrecht
The Netherlands

INNE H. M. BOREL RINKES, MD
Department of Surgery
University Hospital Utrecht
P. O. Box 85500
3508 GA Utrecht
The Netherlands

ALAN J. BRITTEN, MD
Department of Medical Physics
St. George's Hospital
Blackshaw Road
London, SW17 OQT
UK

MARIJKE R. CANNINGA-
VAN DIJK, MD
Department of Pathology
University Hospital Utrecht
P. O. Box 85500
3508 GA Utrecht
The Netherlands

ELLIOT HOWARD-JONES, BA
Finance Directorate
UCLH Trust Hospitals
Mortimer Street
London W1N 8AA
UK

GABRIJELA KOCJAN, FRCPath
Department of Histopathology
Royal Free and University
College Medical School
Rockefeller Building
London W1NE 6JJ
UK

PETER P. VAN RIJK, MD
Department of Nuclear Medicine
University Hospital Utrecht
P. O. Box 85500
3508 GA Utrecht
The Netherlands

WILLEM A. VAN VLOTEN, MD
Department of Dermatology
University Hospital Utrecht
P. O. Box 85500
3508 GA Utrecht
The Netherlands

CHAPTER 1

Sentinel Node Detection and Imaging *

Introduction

The concept of the sentinel node represents a major new opportunity to stratify patients for appropriate surgery in cancer. Present enthusiasm is high judging by the many publications in the peer-reviewed literature, and significant attention is being paid to this subject by editorials in the major medical journals [1–3]. The reports are almost uniformly enthusiastic about the potential of this technique, and guidelines have been published for sentinel node detection in carcinoma of the breast. Patients have become aware of the potential of the technology, and it is not uncommon for patients to inform themselves and request the views of individuals or clinical groups on this new staging procedure. Despite all this enthusiasm, however, there are significant differences in practice relating to almost all aspects of the technology involved. Interestingly, in spite of these differences, in general terms groups are reporting encouraging results. It is therefore useful to review the subject of the detection of the sentinel node, introducing readers to the present areas of uncertainty and providing a critical analysis of the data as they have appeared in the literature.

As can be seen from Table 1, many aspects are being investigated. Several instruments are available for detection of the sentinel node, several radiopharmaceuticals are available for injection, there is controversy as to the injection site, practice varies from single to multiple injections and between large and small volumes of injectate, and there is also considerable variation in the amount of radioactivity administered. With regard to detection, there are groups which advocate external detection with probes and non-imaging, those which combine external detection using a probe with radionuclide gamma camera imaging, those which still advocate the use of blue dye alone or in combination with probe detection, those which have aimed at detection of the sentinel node alone, and those which have

Table 1. Technical issues in sentinel node detection and imaging

What probe?
What tracer?
What injection site?
Single or multiple injection sites?
Large or small volume of injectate?
Massage or no massage of injection site?
How many MBq's?

Which mode of detection is preferable?
- Probe detection only
- Probe detection and imaging
- Blue dye alone or in combination with probe detection
- Sentinel lymph node detection only
- Sentinel lymph node detection and lymphoscintigraphy (imaging)

Which form of imaging is best?
- Dynamic imaging
- Early imaging
- Early and late imaging

What is the most appropriate site of injection?
- Intratumoral
- Peritumoral
- Subdermal
- Subcutaneous

What pathological evidence is required?
- Fine-needle aspiration cytology
- Core cut biopsy
- Use of advanced breast biopsy instrumentation
- Excisional breast biopsy
- Imprint cytology
- Haematoxylin and eosin staining alone
- Cytokeratin immunohistochemistry (e.g. MNF 116)
- Polymerase chain reaction

---

* First published in *Eur J Nucl Med* 26, 1999.

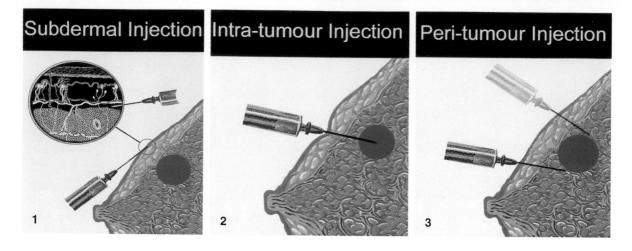

Figs. 1–3. Possible routes for administration of tracer for sentinel node detection. The lymphatic-rich area is seen in Fig. 1

attempted to combine detection of the sentinel node with detection of all lymph nodes in the appropriate lymph basin (lymphoscintigraphy). Furthermore there is significant controversy as to the minimum amount of histopathological evidence which needs to be obtained from the sentinel node.

It is astonishing that groups have used such varying techniques in terms of the delivery of an appropriate radiopharmaceutical to the area of interest (Figs. 1–3). It is well known from the literature that lymphatic tissue is most prevalent in the peripheral layer of the skin, such that a subdermal injection will deliver the tracer to an area rich in lymph vessels. It is also well known that subcutaneous tissue has fewer lymphatic vessels and that direct injection of the tracer into a tumour will consequently entail the administration of an indicator into a high-pressure system. By their nature, tumours have high interstitial and high intercellular pressures, and it is therefore possible that any attempt to administer a tracer directly into a tumour will only lead to leakage of the tracer from the tumour into the peritumoral tissue. There is debate as to the safety of puncturing a tumour directly since there is concern that this may lead to increased seeding of micrometastases from the needle track and puncture of the tumour. There is currently little evidence that this has any effect on the long-term evolution of the tumour and final outcome for a specific patient.

Nevertheless, it would seem appropriate only to perform a direct intratumoral injection if there are clear and overriding advantages – and there is scant evidence in the literature for such advantages.

It is also now clear from the literature that as the sophistication of the methods used to gather pathological evidence from sentinel nodes increases, so there is improved sensitivity of detection of micrometastases. What is not known is the extent to which an ever – increasing sensitivity leads to the detection of a few or even single micrometastases in a lymph node which will fail to develop clinical expression. This issue is raised by an editorial in the *Lancet* [2], where it is almost claimed that all the power of modern histopathological evidence gathering should be aimed not merely at the sentinel node but rather at all the nodes cleared during a surgical axillary lymph node clearance. That this is and probably will remain an entirely impractical proposition is also beyond doubt.

From a legal point of view, radiation protection legislation differs significantly from country to country but in general, a radiopharmaceutical needs to be licensed before it is made available for routine use. The tracers used in Europe for lymphoscintigraphy and sentinel node detection were mostly developed in the early 1970s and were aimed at the imaging of the reticuloendothelial system of the liver, spleen and bone marrow. The properties and overall characteristics of these tracers have therefore not been optimised, in general, for sentinel node detection. There is

Table 2. Inclusion and exclusion criteria employed in our ongoing trial of sentinel node imaging in patients with breast cancer

Eligibility criteria
- All patients with proven carcinoma of the breast on triple assessment (clinical examination, imaging and cytology/tissue diagnosis)
- Palpable and defined non-palpable breast cancer

Exclusion criteria
- Clinical involvement of the axilla
- Pregnancy/lactation
- Multifocal/multicentric carcinomas of the breast
- Previous breast surgery at the same sit

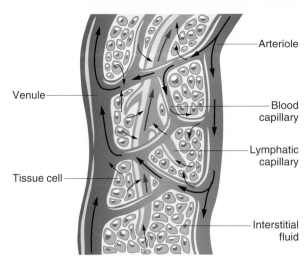

Fig. 4. A representation of lymphatic and blood vessels and the surrounding milieu. (Modified from [27])

significant variability in the particle size of the tracers and ultimately, if this approach is to succeed, an appropriate licenced product will be required in Europe for lymphoscintigraphy in general, for the detection of the sentinel nodes in particular and possibly even for specific applications to specific cancer types.

It is to be emphasised that different results have been obtained with respect to sentinel node detection and imaging in specific patient groups. It is now evident from the literature that poorer results in the detection of the sentinel node in cases of breast cancer are obtained when all lesions are included, when inner quadrant or multicentric lesions are investigated, and when patients are investigated who have already undergone a surgical procedure. Refinement of the indications is in progress in the context of ongoing trials; our own ongoing trial in patients with breast cancer, mirroring that conducted by the Milan group [4], employs the inclusion and exclusion criteria defined in Table 2. In the case of melanoma patients, too, refinement of indications is required.

The Lymphatic System, Lymphoscintigraphy and Sentinel Node Detection

In the past 40 years, a significant body of knowledge has accumulated about the lymphatic system, its dynamics and circulation. Approximately 3 l of lymph flow into the circulation each day, equivalent to 120 ml of lymph flow per hour at rest. Lymphatic flow can increase with exercise by a factor of 10 – 30 and lymphatic channels are seen to contract and relax every 2 – 3 min. The lymphatic

system is hence an extremely dynamic and reactive system. Figures 4 and 5 show diagrammatic representations of a lymph vessel and its relationship with the surrounding milieu. It can be seen that lymph vessels are larger than the surrounding capillaries, and that they are end or terminal vessels with lymph flowing in a single direction determined by valves which ensure the unidirectionality of this flow. Individual lymphatic capillaries are anchored in the surrounding cells by so-called anchoring filaments, which will distend if the surrounding environment is distended (for

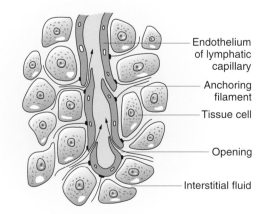

Fig. 5. A representation of a lymphatic capillary. (Modified from [27])

example by the administration of a certain volume of a substance). When particulate substances of an appropriate size are delivered to the interstitial fluid they can traverse the lymphatic capillary endothelium and hence be removed by the lymphatic system towards the first lymph draining nodes.

The first demonstration of lymphatics, by intralymphatic administration of Ethiodol, is accreddited to Kinmonth, in 1952 [5]. The first lympho-auto-radiographic study is attributed to Sherman and Ter-Pogossian [6], who in 1953 demonstrated the concentration of radioactive colloid gold following an interstitial injection in rabbits. At the Middlesex Hospital in 1954 Handley and Thackray, investigating the lymphatic spread of carcinoma of the breast, noted in a series of 150 patients that 10 % were free of axillary disease. In the same year Turner-Warrick performed one of the first lymphoscintigraphic studies in conjunction with blue dye lymph drainage visualisation; his findings were subsequently published in the *Lancet* in 1955 [7].

One of the first lymphoscintigraphic studies in man, investigating the drainage of lymph from the breast to the supplying basins, was performed by Hultborn et al. in 1955, who showed that most of the breast lymph drained to the axilla in these patients [8]. Much more recently, in 1995, Uren et al. investigated the pattern of lymphatic drainage in a group of 34 patients with breast cancer [9]. Drainage to exclusively the axillary node chain was found in 58 % of all cases, to the axillary and internal mammary node chains in 19.4 % of cases, to the axillary, internal mammary and subclavicular node chains in 13 % of cases, to the axillary and infraclavicular node chains in 3.2 % of cases and to the internal mammary node chain in 6.4 % of cases [9]. It is important to underline that this study was carried out with an interstitial administration of antinomy sulphide colloid with very small particle sizes ranging from 3 to 12 nm. A technique with multiple injections was used, surrounding the breast mass and not given subdermally. In this sense the technique was optimised for lymphoscintigraphy but clearly not optimised for the detection of the sentinel node.

Over the years almost every lymphatic basin and region has been demonstrated by lymphoscintigraphy employing a variety of injection techniques and tracers (Table 3), and much useful information has been recorded in the literature. It is evident that we must clearly distinguish between methodology appropriate for the demonstration of all lymph nodes in a particular lymph basin, which we will describe here as lymphoscintigraphy, and techniques suitable for localisation of the first draining lymph node, i.e. the sentinel node. For the former purpose, tracers with a

Table 3. Lymphatic regions demonstrated by lymphoscintigraphy (from Ege GN. Lymphoscintigraphy in oncology. In: Henkin et al., eds. *Nuclear Medicine, vol II.* St. Louis: Mosby; 1996: 1505–1523)

Injection site	Lymph node groups
Dorsum of the foot	Femoral, inguinal, external iliac, para-aortic
Dorsum of the hand	Epitrochlear, axillary, supraclavicular
Mammary, peri-areolar	Axillary, supraclavicular, upper parasternal
Chest wall subcutaneous, subperiosteal	Axillary, supraclavicular, upper parasternal
Subcostal posterior rectus sheath	Diaphragmatic, parasternal, internal mammary ± mediastinal
Buccal mucosa	Jugular
Orbit	Deep cervical
Larynx	Paralaryngeal, superior/inferior jugular
Hepatic capsule	Right parasternal, mediastinal
Splenic capsule	Splenic hilar
Lower oesophagus	Mid-mediastinal, coeliac, upper peri-aortic
Gastric cardia	Coeliac, upper peri-aortic
Peritoneal cavity	Anterior mediastinal
Vulva	Inguinal, external iliac
Rectal	Superior haemorrhoidal, inferior mesenteric, perirectal
Peri-anal, ischiorectal fossa	Internal iliac, presacral, obturator, common iliac, para-aortic
Intraprostatic	Periprostatic, internal iliac
Peritumoral, intracutaneous	Superficial lymphatics at risk

Table 4. Indications for lymphoscintigraphy

Tumour staging
Definition of radiotherapy fields
Evaluation of lymphoedema vs venous oedema
Evaluation of drainage patterns (leaks)
Lymphangiectasia
Chyle stasis

Table 5. Indications for sentinel node detection

Surgical management of:
– Melanoma
– Breast cancer
– Colorectal cancer
– Head and neck cancer
– Penile cancer
– Other

small particle size of less than 20 nm are preferable, whilst for the detection of the sentinel node colloids of larger particle size between 50 and 200 nm, are required. The clinical indications for the two techniques are also different (Tables 4, 5).

Technetium-99m Labelled Colloid Particles

With the report in 1965 by Garzom et al. of a first colloid labelled with the radionuclide technetium-99m [10] a new era began for lymphoscintigraphy. Rapidly, a very large variety of tracers appeared, all labelled with ^{99m}Tc. This radionuclide has ideal characteristics for detection and imaging, having a physical half-life of 6 h and an imaging energy of 140 keV, and in addition is universally available since it can be delivered on a daily basis from a generator. The low cost of ^{99m}Tc per MBq is a further reason why the initial labelling methodology was received with such enthusiasm.

A number of attempts were made to define the optimal characteristics for radiocolloid uptake in lymph nodes and a widely quoted study by Strand and Persson investigated these characteristics in a rabbit model where tracers were injected subcutaneously and bilaterally below the xiphoid process [11]. In general, it was found that the smaller the particle size, the higher was the colloid uptake in parasternal lymph nodes. The study was then extended by the same group, who concluded that the optimum particle size for interstitial lymphoscintigraphy is of the order of tens of nanometres [12]. In a study by Kaplan et al. [13], two ^{99m}Tc-labelled radiopharmaceuticals for lymphoscintigraphy were compared in man (stannous phytate and antimony sulphide). The authors concluded that antimony sulphide was to be preferred since it showed a greater number of internal mammary lymph nodes in patients with breast cancer. Again, in this study a subcostal injection of the radiocolloid was given below the xiphisternum. It is clear that in the 1970s and 1980s the aim of lymphoscintigraphy was to visualise the majority of lymph nodes in a particular lymph basin for staging purposes but also for delineation of lymph flow patterns and better definition of a radiotherapy field. In Table 6 data are compiled from the literature in respect of various radiocolloids and their uptake in parasternal lymph nodes. The data show the huge range of particle sizes and variation in percent uptake at 2 and 5 h following subcostal administration.

Recent in vivo comparisons in man tell a very different story and require reflection. Paganelli et al. investigated three different colloid sizes in a significant number of patients with carcinoma of the breast and determined the number of sentinel nodes detected [14]. The tracer was given subdermally and the methodology optimised for

Table 6. Properties of various radiocolloids, and their uptake in parasternal lymph nodes

Product	Proprietary name	Particle size (nm)	Stability	Uptake % (2 h)	Uptake % (5 h)
mμAA	Microlite	10	Constant	1.5	1.5
μAA	Albucoll	70	Constant	0.3	0.5
Sb$_2$S$_3$	Labelaid	45	Constant	1.1	1.7
(Sn)S	Hepato	90	Constant	0.3	0.4
(Re)S		360, 60	Constant	0.3	1.3
μAA	AlbuRES	250	Constant	0.6	0.7
Sulphur	In-house	600	Variable	0.2	–

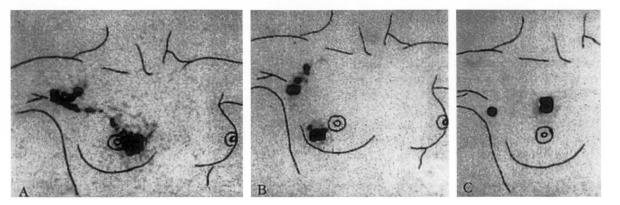

Fig. 6 and Table 7. The relationship between colloid particle size and number of sentinel nodes imaged. The smaller the particles, the greater the number of nodes imaged. (From Paganelli et al., *Q J Nucl Med* 1998; 42: 49–53)

Table 7

Size of Tracer (nm)	Positive Patients	No. of nodes
< 50	29/30	1–5
< 80	26/30	1–4
< 200 < 1000	155/155	1–2

sentinel node imaging and detection. Figure 6 and Table 7 summarise the main findings. From this it can be seen that the tracers with smaller particle sizes resulted in the visualisation of a greater number of lymph nodes, paradoxically rendering more difficult the imaging and external detection of the sentinel node. Best results were obtained with the larger particle size colloids.

In a study by Glass et al. published in 1998 the kinetics of three lymphoscintigraphic agents were investigated in patients with cutaneous melanoma [15]. Whilst all agents were passed through a similar sized filter (200 nm) it became clear that for sentinel node imaging, detection at 30 min is more appropriate than late imaging. Having passed the three agents through a similar sized filter, there were no significant differences in the quality of nodal visualisation or the half-times of tracer washout from these nodes.

Briefly summarising, then, it can be stated (Tables 8, 9) that there is a need to identify an ideal colloid for sentinel node visualisation, which will clearly be different from a particulate tracer optimised for the visualisation of all lymph nodes. It will be important that the exact range of particle sizes is known, that the product is stable on storage, that it is labelled with ^{99m}Tc and that it contains particles of an average size of the order of 80–200 nm. In fact the study by Paganelli et al. [14], where the authors quote a particle size range of 200–1000, is likely to have been conducted with a range of particles not exceeding 400 nm (personal observations).

Table 8. Characteristics of the ideal colloid

Licensed product
Narrow particle size range
^{99m}Tc label
Stable on storage
Lymph channel transport
Rapid transport
Retention in sentinel node
Stable in blood (no shrinkage or growth)

Table 9. Fate of colloids according to particle size

Particle size	Fate
Few nm	Exchange through blood capillaries
Tens of nm	Absorbed into lymph capillaries
Hundreds of nm	Trapped in interstitial space
Large particles	Do not migrate

Probe Selection

Once a radiopharmaceutical is administered, the passage of the tracer through the lymphatic system can be recorded fairly accurately. Imaging devices such as the conventional Anger gamma camera are ideally suited to record the early tracking of the tracer into the lymphatic vessels, given that they permit rapid imaging over short intervals of time. Early imaging, commencing immediately after administration of the tracer, will give a prompt indication of the progress of the radiocolloid from the administered site. It will also provide an early warning, should the tracer fail to migrate. External probes are non-imaging detectors which can be optimised for intra-operative use. They hence allow a specific signal to be picked up from a focussed site within the body where the greatest concentration of tracer is encountered. With the renewed interest in sentinel node detection, probe technology has changed rapidly over the past few years, mainly in order to optimise portability, ease of use and signal detection.

In determining the most appropriate probe, consideration is usually given to sensitivity (number of counts detected per unit of time per area detector), resolution (the minimum distance between two signals which can be separated with sufficient statistical certainty), energy resolution (the ability of the probe to distinguish degraded from non-degraded radiation), collimation (the ability of the detector to pick up a signal from a circumscribed volume of tissue to be investigated), and other features such as the overall ergonomics and design of the probe, the ease of perioperative use, facilities for use in a sterile environment and cost. Probe manufacturers are listed in Table 10.

A recent paper by Tiourina et al. [16] reviews the main characteristics of a number of probes available for sentinel lymph node detection. It is noteworthy that these characteristics vary significantly. Thus the resolution of probes may vary by a factor of 4, the transmission of signal through the shielding surrounding the detector may vary by a factor as great as 40 and the detection sensitivity of the probes in air or water may also vary by a factor of the order of 20! The reader is referred to the work of Tiourina et al. for a more detailed technical assessment.

Table 10. Examples of probe types and manufacturers

USSC Navigator
Neoprobe 1500, 2000
(C-Trak) Care Wise
Eurorad (Gammed)
ScintiProbe MR 100-Pol.hi.tech.

Carcinoma of the Breast

Breast cancer is a major disease. The 5-year survival rate is not much better than 85% for all stages. Localised disease has a 5-year survival rate of the order of 96%, dropping to 75% with regional spread and to 20% with distant spread. It is also known that axillary lymph node-positive patients are more likely to develop distant metastases, that axillary lymph node-positive patients die earlier and that postoperative adjuvant chemotherapy significantly reduces the risk of distant disease and dissemination. For all these reasons knowledge of the status of the sentinel lymph node chain is a most important prognostic factor and hence crucial for the appropriate management of these patients.

The theoretical basis for sentinel node detection in carcinoma of the breast is set out in Table 11. It is assumed that the first regional lymph node which drains lymph from a primary tumour is the first node to receive the seeding of lymph-borne metastatic cells. A survey of the literature does appear to indicate that tumour cells disseminate fairly sequentially and that so-called skip metastases are only rarely encountered.

There are two fundamental concepts which, however, are still the cause of much controversy. It has been stated (*Lancet* 1998) that the sentinel node concept is too Halstedian in nature. Tumours do not evolve and disseminate into local, regional and distant metastases in an orderly fashion (Figs. 7, 8). Indeed, most tumour biologists would lead us to believe that tumours have seeded distally at the time of clinical presentation or manifestation. This debate will continue in the literature but it is fair to state that advocates of sentinel node scintigraphy and detection

Table 11. Theoretical basis for sentinel node detection

Lymph flow is orderly and predictable
Tumour cells disseminate sequentially
The sentinel or "first" lymph node is the first node encountered by tumour cells
Sentinel node status predicts distant basin status
Patients present with earlier stage of disease
Basin involvement is less frequent
Surgery can be targeted to the appropriate population

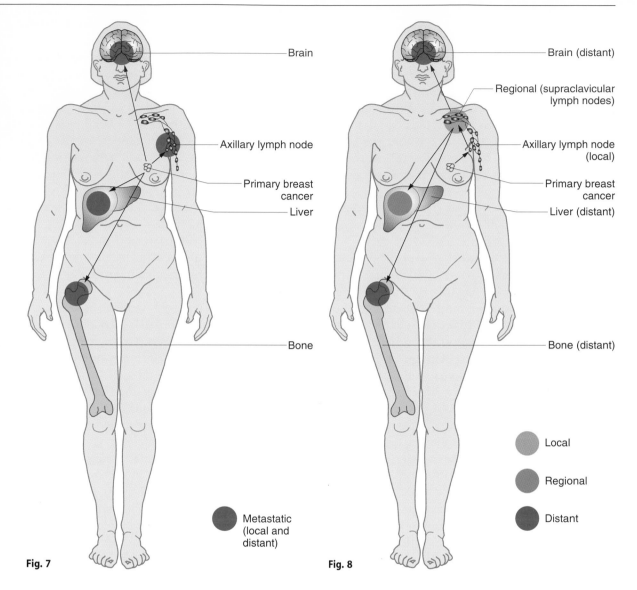

Fig. 7

Fig. 8

Figs. 7 and 8. A representation of the metastatic spread of breast cancer: a random progression (17) or an orderly progression (18). (Modified from [28])

need to be aware of the possible pitfalls in this approach.

From a surgical management point of view, however, it is also clear that a significant number of patients who undergo axillary lymph node clearance do endure pain and significant side-effects, with no apparent benefit. Between 70% and 80% of breast cancer patients referred to a modern practice will have completely negative surgical axillary lymph node exploration, and 3%–12% of patients do develop limiting lymphoedema with

the associated morbidity. The additional costs of surgical exploration of the axilla must also be taken into account. On the other hand, an important study by Turner et al. (1997) provides ample evidence supporting the sentinel node hypothesis for breast carcinoma [17]. If H & E staining and immunohistochemistry indicate that the sentinel node is not involved, then the probability of non-sentinel node involvement is less than 0.1% (the false-negative rate was 0.97%, i.e. 1 patient in 103).

A thesis by B. A. E. Kapteijn on biopsy of the sentinel node in melanoma, penile carcinoma and breast carcinoma (submitted to the Netherlands Cancer Institute, 1997) documents that successful

Table 12. Results of sentinel node biopsy in breast carcinoma (data compiled by B.A.E. Kapteijn, The Netherlands Cancer Institute, 1997)

Author (year) in vivo/ ex vivo	No. of patients	Injection technique (peri/ intra)	PBD/ tracer	Size of primary tumour	Identifi- cation rate (%)	Metastases (%)	Remarks
Krag (1993), in vivo	22	Peri	Tracer	Not given	82	39	In 2 cases of posi- tive lymph nodes, no SN found
Giuliano (1994), in vivo	174	Intra	PBD	Tis: 15 mm T1: 104 mm >T2: 55 mm	66	32	FN = 5
Giuliano (1995), in vivo	134 ALND 162 SLND	Intra	PBD	Median: 1.5 cm	100	29 42	FN rate not given
Uren (1995), in vivo	34 (3: + ALND)	Peri	Tracer PBD (3)	Not given	100	67	FN rate = 0% LS performed
Schneebaum (1996), in vivo	15	Not given	Tracer + PBD	Not given	87	20	FN = 1 LS performed
Meijer (1996), in vivo	30	Peri	Tracer	18 < 2 cm	100	32	FN = 0 LS performed (2 cases; no SN)
Kapteijn (1996), ex vivo	30	Intra	PBD	Mean: 2.9 cm	87	38	FN = 0
Albertini (1996)	62	Peri	Tracer/ PBD	Mean: 2.2 cm	92	32	FN = 0 LS performed

SN, Sentinel node; PBD, blue dye; FN, false-negative; ALND, axillary lymphadenectomy; SLND, sentinel lymph node dissection; LS, lymphoscintigraphy.

localisation of the sentinel node in breast carcinoma has been possible since 1993. However, there has been significant variability in results and methodological practice, as shown by Table 12.

A recent meta-analysis of 821 patients with carcinoma of the breast reported an overall success rate of 93.5% for localisation of the sentinel node. This is very similar to the 92% rate reported by Albertini et al. in 1996 with reference to 62 patients [18]. Albertini et al. also documented an absence of skip metastases and the fact that in 67% of all patients with a positive sentinel node, this was the only site of disease. Veronesi et al., reporting in the *Lancet* in 1997, investigated 163 patients and reported 97.5% accuracy in the prediction of the lymph node status! In 95% of patients there was concordance between a negative sentinel node and negative status of the axillary nodes. Albertini et al. [18] stated that "the

beauty of lymphatic mapping is that it allows the surgeon to give the pathologist one or two sentinel nodes to perform a more detailed examination". They also considered that the results suggest that sentinel node biopsy using a gamma probe can identify negative axillary nodes with high accuracy [4].

Borgstein, reporting in 1998 on 130 patients, demonstrated the sentinel node in 89% of cases; the failure rate was significant in patients submitted to previous excision biopsy (36%) and there was a small failure rate (4%) when the tumour was palpable in situ. Biopsy of the sentinel node was 98% accurate for the prediction of nodal metastases [3]. Also in 1998, Cox et al. showed successful identification of the sentinel node in 94% of 466 patients [19].

Clearly these data, derived from several studies with large samples, give credence to the sentinel node concept and strongly point to the need for a large multicentre trial which would ultimately determine the appropriate clinical indications for this methodology and its impact on the surgical management of patients presenting with carcinoma of the breast.

Melanoma

Approximately 80 million cases of melanoma have been reported in Europe. The incidence appears to be increasing, with the 5-year survival heavily dependent on tumour thickness. For tumours of less than 1.5 mm thickness and without metastases, survival is greater than 90%; for tumours greater than 4 mm thickness, survival drops to 50%, and it falls even further, to 10%, when patients present with distant metastases. Most melanomas (65%) are of the superficial spreading type; nodular melanoma accounts for 25% of cases, lentigo maligna melanoma for 5% and acrolentiginous melanoma for 5%.

Very significant experience has been obtained with regard to sentinel node detection in melanoma. Again from the data compiled by Kapteijn (Table 13) it can be seen that many studies have been carried out since the early investigations by Morton et al. in 1992 [20]. A review article by Singluff et al. in 1994 on the surgical management of regional lymph nodes in 4682 patients offers interesting background information [21]. Although in this particular analysis lymphoscintigraphy was performed only in a minority of patients, the authors concluded that lymphoscintigraphy is probably the best way to identify basins draining a specific area of the skin. It was also stated that the number of basins identified by this methodology may overestimate the number of basins in which nodal metastases acquire clinical relevance. Clearly the concept of the sentinel node was set to emerge. In the same year Reintgen et al. published an important study on the orderly progression of melanoma and nodal metastases (Figs. 9, 10). Forty-two patients were investigated, of whom 34 had histologically negative sentinel

Table 13. Results of sentinel node biopsy in melanoma (data compiled by B.A.E. Kapteijn, The Netherlands Cancer Institute, 1997)

Author (year)	No. of patients	Breslow thickness	Identification of sentinel node (%)	Medhod (BD/GDP)	Metastases (% patients)	False-negative rate (%)
Morton (1992)	223	CS-I[a]	82	BD	21	1
Morton (1994)	72	68: >0.65 mm 2: <0.65 mm 2: unknown	90	BD	15	0
Lingham (1994)	15	Mean: 3.75 mm (range 1.5–8.1)	100	BD	27	0
Thompson (1995)	118	111: >1.5 mm 7: <1.5 mm	87	BD	23	0
Krag (1995)	121	109: >0.75 <4 mm 11: >4 mm 1: unknown	98	GDP: 77 BD + GDP: 44	12	0
Abertini (1996)	106	Mean: 2.24 mm (>0.75 mm)	96	GDP + BD	15	0
Mudun (1996)	25	3: <1.5 mm 18: >1.5 <4 mm 4: >4 mm	100	GDP	24	Not given
Karakousis (1995)	55	>1 mm	93	BD	24	Not given
Kapteijn (1995)	110	>1 mm	99.5	GDP+BD	23	2.7

[a] Clinical stage I: clinically localised melanoma; no palpable lymph nodes.
BD, Blue dye; GDP, gamma detection probe.

Figs. 9 and 10.
The influence of Breslow thickness on survival and the relationship of the positivity of PCR with tumour thickness for melanoma at presentation. (From Reintgen et al., *Ann Surg* 1997; 225: 1–14)

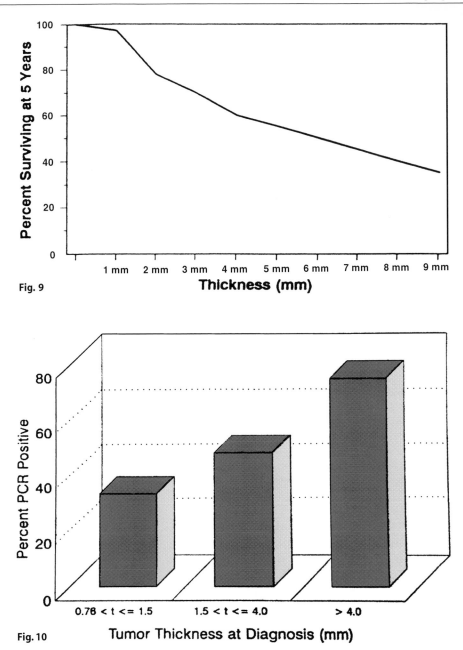

Fig. 9

Fig. 10

nodes, with the remainder of the nodes in the basin also being negative. No skip metastases were documented. The authors concluded that nodal metastases from cutaneous melanoma are not random events. Sentinel nodes in the lymphatic basins could be mapped and identified individually, and these were shown to contain the first evidence of melanoma metastases. The authors concluded that this information could be used to revolutionise melanoma care [22].

In 1996 Albertini et al. reported on 106 consecutive patients, comparing the sentinel node detection technique with vital blue dye mapping. Whilst the blue dye staining identified 69.5% of sentinel nodes, radioisotope detection allowed for the identification of 83.5%. When combined, these techniques detected 96% of the sentinel nodes [23].

The following year Leong et al. reported their results obtained in 163 patients. The success rate for detection of the sentinel node was 98%, the frequency of microscopic metastatic melanoma involving the sentinel node was 18.4%, and 27.3% of sentinel nodes were detected in the absence of blue dye! The authors concluded that gamma probe-guided resection would minimise the extent of lymph node dissection [24].

A study by Joseph et al. in 1998 looked at 83 melanoma patients with a positive sentinel node, among a total of 600 stage 1–2 patients. The sentinel node was positive in 30% of patients with a tumour thickness greater than 4 mm, 18% with a tumour thickness between 1.5 and 4 mm, 7% with a tumour thickness between 1.0 and 1.5 mm and 0% with a tumour thickness of less than 0.76 mm [25].

Cascinelli et al., publishing in the *Lancet* in 1998, confirmed that elective regional node dissection is not efficacious, that the dissection of clinically undetectable nodal metastases will lead to higher long-term survival, that the detection of the sentinel node will help the selection of patients with occult disease who will benefit from regional node dissection and that even Breslow thickness appears to be less important when adjusted by the status of regional lymph nodes [26].

Conclusion

A vast amount of literature has now been published relating to the detection of the sentinel node and its impact on the surgical management of cancer. Whilst most data have been collated from patients suffering from carcinoma of the breast or skin (melanoma), there is increasing interest in other areas such as head and neck cancer, colorectal cancer and penile cancer.

It does appear that the relatively new technique of detection of the sentinel node (as opposed to lymphoscintigraphy) is highly successful and accurate and that the correlation between histological involvement of this node and that of distant basins is very promising indeed. There is sufficient evidence in the literature to affirm that the time has come for a detailed cost-benefit analysis of these techniques in large multicentre trials, and there is hope that this methodology may become part of the routine surgical management of large numbers of patients. However, there is

evident scope for improvement of the technology involved and refinement of protocols.

Currently it can be stated that detection of the sentinel node is highly accurate at least in the context of carcinoma of the breast and melanoma, that there is a rapidly increasing database population, and that training programmes relevant to multi-disciplinary teams need to be developed for this methodology, with emphasis on standardisation of tracer and techniques, improved design of detector technology and patient education.

References

1. Dixon M. Sentinel node biopsy in breast cancer. *Br Med J* 1998; 317:295–296
2. della Rovere G, Bird PA. Sentinel-lymph-node in breast cancer. *Lancet* 1998; 352:421–422
3. Borgstein PJ. SLN biopsy in breast cancer: guidelines and pitfalls of lymphoscintigraphy and gamma probe detection. *J Am Coll Surg* 1998; 186:275–283
4. Veronesi U, Paganelli G, Galimberti V, Viale G, Zurrida ST, Bodeni N, Costa A, Chicco C, Geraghty JG, Luine A, Sacchini V, Veronesi P. Sentinel-node biopsy to avoid axillary dissection in breast cancer with clinicaly negative lymph-nodes. *Lancet* 1997; 349:1864–1867
5. Kinmonth JB. Lymphangiogram in man: method outlining lymphatic trunks and operation. *Clin Sci* 1952; 11:13–20
6. Sherman A, Ter-Pogossian M. Lymph node concentration of radioactive colloid gold following insterstitial injection. *Cancer* 1953; 6:1238–1240
7. Turner-Warrick R. The demonstration of lymphatic vessels. *Lancet* 1955; 1:1371
8. Hultborn KA, Larsson LG, Ragnhult I. The lymph drainage from the breast to the axillary and parasternal lymph node: studied with the help of Au-198. *Acta Radiol* 1955; 43:52–64
9. Uren RF, Howman-Giles RB, Thompson JF, Malouf D, Ramsey-Stewart G, Niesche FW, Renwick SB. Mammary lymphoscintigraphy in breast cancer. *J Nucl Med* 1995; 36:1775–1780
10. Garzom OL, Palcos MC, Radicella R. Technetium-99m labelled colloid. *Int J Appl Radiat Isotopes* 1965; 16:613
11. Strand S-E, Persson DRR. Quantitative lymphoscintigraphy. I. Basic concepts for optimal uptake of radiocolloids in the parasternal lymph nodes of rabbits. *J Nucl Med* 1979; 1038–1046
12. Bergqvist L, Srand SE, Persson B, Hafstrom L, Jonsson PE. Dosimetry in lymphoscintigraphy of Tc-99m antimony sulfide colloid. *J Nucl Med* 1982; 23:698–705
13. Kaplan WD, Davies MA, Rose CHN. A comparison of two technetium-99m labelled radiopharmaceuticals for lymphoscintigraphy: concise communication. *J Nucl Med* 1979; 20:933–937
14. Paganelli G, Chicco C, Cremonesi M, Prisco G, Calza P, Luini A, Zucali P, Veronesi U. Optimised sentinel node scintigraphy in breast cancer. *Q J Nucl Med* 1998; 42:49–53

15. Glass EC, Essner R, Morton DL. Kinetics of three lymphoscintigraphic agents in patients with cutaneous melanoma. *J Nucl Med* 1998; 39:1185–1190

16. Tiourina T, Arends B, Huysmans D, Rutten H, Lemaire B, Muller S. Evaluation of surgical gamma probes for radioguided sentinel node localisation. *Eur J Nucl Med* 1998; 25:1224–1231

17. Turner RR, Ollila DW, Krasne DL, Giuliano AE. Histopathological validation of the sentinel lymph node hypothesis for breast carcinoma. *Ann Surg* 1997; 226:271–278

18. Albertini JJ, Lyman GH, Cox C, Yeatman T, Balducci L, Ku N, Shivers S, Berman C, Wells K, Rapaport D, Shons A, Horton J, Greenberg H, Nicosia S, Clark R, Cantor A, Reintgen DS. Lymphatic mapping and sentinel node biopsy in the patient with breast cancer. *J Am Med Assoc* 1996; 276:1818–1822

19. Cox CE, Pendas S, Cox JM, Joseph E, Shons AR, Yeatman T, Ku NN, Lyman GH, Berman C, Haddad F, Reintgen DS. Guidelines for SN biopsy and lymphatic mapping of patients with breast cancer. *Ann Surg* 1998; 227:645–653

20. Morton DL, Wen D-R, Wong GH, et al. Technical details of intra-operative lymphatic mapping for early stage melanoma. *Arch Surg* 1992; 127:392–399

21. Slingluff, CL Jr., Stidham KR, Ricci WM, Stanley WE, Seigler HF. Surgical management of regional lymph nodes in patients with melanoma. Experience with 4,682 patients. *Ann Surg* 1994; 219:120–130

22. Reintgen D, Cruse CW, Wells K, Berman C, Fenske N, Glass F, Schroer K, Heller R, Ross M, Lyman G, Cox C, Rapaport D, Seigler HF, Balch C. The orderly progression of melanoma nodal metastases. *Ann Surg* 1994; 220:759–767

23. Albertini JJ, Cruse CW, Rapaport D, Wells K, Ross M, DeConti R, Berman CG, Jared K, Messina J, Lyman G, Glass F, Fenske N, Reintgen DS. Intraoperative radiolymphoscintigraphy improves sentinel lymph node identification for patients with melanoma. *Ann Surg* 1996; 223:217–224

24. Leong SPL, Steinmetz I, Habib FA, McMillan A, Gans JZ, Allen RE Jr, Morita E, El-Kadi M, Epstein HD, Kashani-Sabet M, Sagebiel RW. Optimal selective sentinel lymph node dissection in primary malignant melanoma. *Arch Surg* 1998; 132:666–673

25. Joseph E, Brobeil A, Glass F, Glass J, Messina J, DeConti R, Cruse CW, Rapaport DP, Berman C, Fenske N, Reintgen DS. Results of complete lymph node dissection in 83 melanoma patients with positive SLN. *Ann Surg Oncol* 1998; 5:119–125

26. Cascinelli N, Morabito A, Santinami M, MacKie RM, Belli F. Immediate or delayed dissection of regional nodes in patients with melanoma of the trunk: a randomised trial. WHO Melanoma Programme. *Lancet* 1998; 351:793–796

27. Tortora GJ, Reynold S, Grabowski S. *Principles of anatomy and physiology, 8th edn.* Addison Wesley Longman, 1996

28. Hayes DF. *Atlas of breast cancer.* Mosby, 1993

CHAPTER 2

Radiopharmaceuticals

A radiopharmaceutical is a specific compound which has been labelled with a small amount of a radionuclide in order to allow this product to be detected externally once given parenterally to a patient. Both the substance to be labelled and the radioactive nuclide are usually used in such small amounts that no pharmacological effect ensues upon administration to the patient. Often the designations "tracer" and "trace amounts" are employed since the chemical quantities which are labelled are in the order of a millionth of a gram. External detection of the signal emitted by the radiopharmaceutical allows the tracer to be recorded either by a probe (such as for the peroperative detection of the sentinel node) or by an imaging device, such as the Anger gamma camera. The latter is then used to obtain an image of the distribution of the tracer in a specific region of the body. In the case of visualisation of the lymphatic pathways, the word "lymphoscintigraphy" is most appropriately used.

In conventional and routine nuclear medicine applications the radionuclide most often used for labelling purposes is technetium-99m (^{99m}Tc). It is now universally available for daily use at a very economic price. ^{99m}Tc is produced indirectly either by the neutron irradiation of molybdenum-98 or as a fission product of uranium-235. ^{99m}Tc generators are supplied by a variety of commercial manufacturers, usually on a once a week basis. The generator consists of molybdenum-99 adsorbed on an alumina column. Through fission, carrier-free molybdenum-99 is obtained, such that large quantities of the nuclide can be adsorbed onto a rather small alumina column. The generator can be eluted daily with saline, and sterile and pyrogen-free ^{99m}Tc in the form of pertechnetate is obtained. In the larger radiopharmacies many hundreds of individual doses can be prepared for individual patient use.

Technetium-99m pertechnetate (^{99m}TcO$_4^-$) is a relatively stable form (VII) of technetium. Alone it will usually not bind to other compounds and so it is most often reduced by reducing agents, such as stannous chloride, to more positively charged technetium species (III to VI) much more amenable to chemical reactions with a host of other compounds. An exception to this important rule is ^{99m}Tc sulphur colloid, which seems to have the Tc(VII) oxidation state. Since technetium sulphide is relatively insoluble, it allows ^{99m}Tc to remain in the VII state of oxidation. Stabilising agents such as gelatin and albumin are often used.

Radiopharmaceuticals for Lymph Node Detection and Lymphoscintigraphy

For the purposes of lymph node detection and lymphoscintigraphy, labelled colloids seem to be most appropriate. Indeed, many different labelled radiopharmaceuticals are available for lymphoscintigraphy, and a brief summary of these has already been provided in Chap. 1.

To some extent the choice of colloid will depend on the purpose of the study and there are clearly a number of issues which merit consideration. Ultimately, however, in this increasingly regulatory environment only nationally registered radiopharmaceuticals can be used routinely in patients. This is already limiting the choices and possibilities. Registration of new radiopharmaceuticals is very costly and is hampering the development of the field as a whole. Most of the present compounds were manufactured for the purpose of imaging liver, spleen and bone marrow, at a time when neither diagnostic ultrasound nor computed X-ray tomography was available for the non-invasive imaging of these organs. It is important to remember this in view of what has been stated above and in understanding the optimisation which these compounds have undergone for the purpose of visualisation of the reticuloendothelial system in man. These tracers were given intravenously; rapid uptake by Kupffer cells was aimed at, with a rapidly falling blood clearance of the labelled tracers.

Put in rather general terms, labelled colloids must be prepared in a reproducible manner, be and remain stable once labelled, have a reasonable shelf life and have a well-defined particle size range. This is easier said than achieved. It is important to appreciate that different particle sizes will influence the methodology and results to be gained. When administered in the intercellular space, smaller particles will migrate much more rapidly from the injection site and will require rapid monitoring, both for imaging and for external probe detection. Larger particles will migrate much more slowly and will require late imaging records and external probe detection. At present, there is no clear consensus as to an optimal particle size for the detection of the sentinel node and it is our contention that different particle sizes may need to be used for lymphoscintigraphy (namely the imaging of all lymph nodes from one particular basin) and for the detection of the few sentinel nodes relevant in a particular cancer. It may even turn out that for melanoma or breast carcinoma better results can be achieved with one tracer than with another. Sizing particles from different colloids may involve practical methodologies such as the use of filters or more advanced technology such as the electron microscope, X-ray fluorescence or gel chromatography. An excellent review of this subject is to be found in an article published by Bergqvist et al. (1983). Early work on this topic was also performed by Frier et al. (1981), Warbick et al. (1977) and Persson (1970).

The trapping of particles by lymph nodes has always been considered to occur as a result of macrophage activity and phagocytosis. Whilst particle size is relevant, so are the particle numbers and the charge of the particle. When in contact with sera particles may change in size;

this appears to happen with sulphur colloid particles and to a lesser extent with albumin particles. Temperature, pH and length of the manufacturing process all influence the distribution of the particle sizes obtained. Alazraki et al. (1997) found major variations in the labelling yield of sulphur colloid particles. When a kit was heated for 10 min and allowed to cool for 5 min, a higher radiochemical purity of the end product was obtained. The use of a reduced heating time resulted in a significant increase in the percentage of particles smaller than 400 nm. With increased heating time a significant decrease in the percentage of smaller particles was seen. There was also a difference when a ^{99m}Tc generator was used fresh or when older eluates from the generator were used for the labelling procedure. In fact for sulphur colloid Alazraki recommends the use of a 3-min rather than a 5-min heating protocol, and the use of an older rather than a fresher generator eluate.

From Table 6 in Chap. 1 one can see the significant variation in particle size. It is necessary to emphasise that most of the literature describing the distribution of these labelled colloids in animal experiments or in man has referred to data obtained with injection techniques not optimised for the detection of the sentinel node. So whilst there is a significant amount of literature which discusses the impact of injection techniques, particle size and the visualisation of lymph node chains, specific studies for the investigation of these factors in the detection of the sentinel node are still needed. Caution needs to be exercised when extrapolating from animal data on particle migration and uptake ratios in specific nodal chains after subcutaneous administration in the xiphoid area, with the patterns to be expected when the same tracers are given, for example, subdermally in the human breast.

From own observations it is also clear that with certain types of preparations, particle sizes may vary considerably from batch to batch. In recent experiments we found between – batch variations of the order of a factor of 4 for the same preparation from the same manufacturer. It is vital that batch quality control of the preparations is available in order to reduce these variations, which will clearly impact on practice and results. Whilst for lymphoscintigraphy average particle sizes of the order of 50–80 nm may be favoured, for the detection of the sentinel node it may be preferable to aim for a preparation of between 100 and 200 nm. Larger particle sizes will migrate slowly and might lead to inferior data collection.

A study specifically designed to clarify these issues is needed and probably in progress, despite the inherent difficulties to be overcome when comparing more than one tracer in man (given the expected variability to be encountered when lymph nodes are to be detected). We have already referred to the study of Paganelli et al. (1998) in Chapt. 1, where different migration patterns were shown when colloids of different size were used for the detection of the sentinel node in patients with carcinoma of the breast. What is not known is the exact range of the distribution of the particle size used in this study.

Typical Preparations

■ *Nanocoll* (manufacturer: Sorin Biomedica Diagnostics, Italy). This preparation contains 0.5 mg of human serum albumin with 95% of labelled particles below 80 nm.

■ *Albu-Res* (manufacturer: Sorin Biomedica Diagnostics, Italy). This preparation contains 2.5 mg of human serum albumin with 90% of the labelled particles between 200 and 1000 nm.

■ *Nanocis* (manufacturer: CIS bio International, France). This preparation contains colloidal rhenium sulphide (0.48 mg) with an average particle size range of 3–15 nm.

■ *Microlite* (manufacturer: DuPont, USA). A preparation of 1 mg of human serum albumin with an average particle size of 10 nm.

■ *Sulphur Colloid* (manufacturer: CIS-US). This preparation is available in the USA; depending on the labelling protocol, the labelled particles are between 40 and 1000 nm.

■ *Antimony Sulfide Colloid*. This preparation has been used mostly in Australia and has a very small particle size composition, 5–15 nm.

■ *Gold-198*. This was the first tracer to be used for lymphoscintigraphy. It has a good and uniform particle size range of about 5 nm. It is no longer in use owing to the excessive radiation dose delivered to the target organs.

■ *Other Compounds*. The other compounds that have been tried out include ^{99m}Tc dextran with a molecular weight of 100000 (lower molecular weight dextran exhibits capillary transport) (Henze et al. 1982) and ^{99m}Tc-labelled human serum albumin (Nawaz et al. 1985). Recently, ^{99m}Tc-labelled polyclonal human immunoglobulin has also been tested for lymphoscintigraphy and lymph flow measurements (Svensson et al. 1998).

It may well be that different surgical units will opt for one preparation rather than another once the implications of particle size are fully appreciated. For example, if a patient is to be imaged on one day and operated on the following day, larger colloids may be more appropriate than if the aim is to administer the colloid on the same day as the operation and the external detection of the sentinel node. Furthermore, it may be that in some pathologies it is more important also to visualise the flow of lymph rather than just the sentinel node; again, this could impact on choice. It has already been shown that smaller particles will detect a greater number of lymph nodes and that this approach may be more useful in one pathology than in another.

Conclusion

Most labelled colloids were developed by the radiopharmaceutical industry in the early 1970s for liver, spleen and bone marrow scintigraphy. The size of the colloidal particles was optimised such that, once given intravenously, the pulmonary capillary bed could be bypassed and the particles would then be trapped by the reticuloendothelial system.

The term "colloids" was usually reserved for particle sizes below 300–400 nm. The term "microaggregate" was reserved for particle sizes of 500–3000 nm and the term "macroaggregate" for particle sizes greater than 5000 nm. It is not easy to determine the particle size of a colloid by conventional means since colloidal particles are usually not seen in the optical microscope. Electron microscopy is often used, as is gel chromatography. A practical approach allows for the use of filters of different pore size in order to remove larger particles from a preparation and thus obtain a narrower particle size range.

Human serum albumin preparations are mostly used in Europe and are available from several manufacturers. Most kits require optimisation for reproducible results to be obtained.

It is to be expected that manufacturers will optimise new kits for the non-invasive detection of the sentinel node, with improved stability of the preparations. The interest generated by these new clinical applications of the radioactive tracer method will justify the effort and cost necessary to achieve the desired outcome. In view of the inherent difficulties in keeping a stable particle size it may well be that other types of particulate compounds will be developed – for example recent work suggests that ^{99m}Tc-labelled liposomes could represent a step forward in this field. ^{99m}Tc-labelled liposomes with an average size of greater than 100 nm migrate somewhat less from the injection site than liposomes with an average size of less than 100 nm (Phillips et al. 1998).

References

1. Bergqvist L, Strand SE, Persson RR. Particle sizing and biokinetics of interstitial lymphoscintigraphic agents. *Semin Nucl Med* 1983; XIII:9–19
2. Frier M, Griffiths P, Ramsey A. The physical and chemical characteristics of sulphur colloids. *Eur J Nucl Med* 1981; 6:255–260
3. Warbick A, Ege GN, Henkelman RM, Maier G, Lyster DM. An evaluation of radiocolloid sizing techniques. *J Nucl Med* 1977; 18:827–834
4. Persson RBR, Naversten Y. Technetium 99m sulfide colloid preparation for scintigraphy of the recticulo-endothelial system. *Acta Radiol Ther Phys Biol* 1970; 9:567–576
5. Alazraki NP, Eshima D, Eshima LA, Herda St C, Murray DR, Vansant JP, Taylor AT. Lymphoscintigraphy, the sentinel node concept and the intraoperative gamma probe in melanoma, breast cancer and other potential cancers. *Semin Nucl Med* 1997; XXVII:55–68
6. Paganelli G, Chicco C, Cremonesi M, Prisco G, Calza P, Luini A, Zucali P, Veronesi U. Optimised sentinel node scintigaphy in breast cancer. *Q J Nucl Med* 1998; 42:49–53
7. Henze E, Schelbert HR, Collins JD, Barrio JRE, Bennett LR. Lymphoscintigraphy with Tc-99m dextran. *J Nucl Med* 1982; 23:923–929
8. Nawaz K, Hamad M, Sadek S, Audeli M, Higazi E, Eklof B, Abdel-Dayem HM. Lymphoscintigraphy in peripheral lymphedema using technetium-labelled human serum albumin: normal and abnormal patterns. *Lymphology* 1985; 18:729–735
9. Svensson W, Glass DM, Bradley D, Peters AM. Lymphoscintigraphy with Tc-99m polyclonal immunoglobulin. *Eur J Nucl Med* (in Press)
10. Phillips WT, Andrews T, Liu HL, Klipper R, Laundry A, Goins B. Evaluation of Tc-99m labeled liposomes versus Tc-99m sulfur colloid and Tc-99m human serum albumin for lymphoscintigraphy in a rabbit model. *J Nucl Med* 1989; 39:314P–315P

CHAPTER 3

Radiation Detectors

Intra-operative Radiation Detectors

Radiation detectors have been used intra-operatively to identify and localise pathology for nearly 50 years, and a number of clinical applications are documented in the published literature.

Clinical Applications

Radiation detection systems were first used intra-operatively in 1949, when Selverstone and associates successfully used narrow-bore Geiger-Müller needle probes to detect the uptake of sodium phosphate incorporating the beta-emitting radionuclide phosphorus-32 in a range of cerebral tumours [1]. The physical characteristics for ^{32}P and other radionuclides discussed in this section are listed in Table 1.

Harris [2] and subsequently Morris and colleagues [3] developed a miniaturised CsI(Tl) scintillation probe to assist in the removal of occult thyroid cancer through detection of its uptake of either iodine-131 or iodine-125. Lennquist and co-workers have also used this technique to remove residual tissue at thyroidectomy, successfully avoiding the need for postoperative radio-iodine ablation in more than half of those patients demonstrating a residual uptake of iodine [4, 5].

Radiodetection probes have also been used to ensure the complete resection of osteoid osteoma, utilising its avidity for technetium-99m labelled phosphonate tracers. Harvey and Lancaster were the first to investigate this technique, and they designed a scintillation detector incorporating a fibre-optic light guide to aid its miniaturisation [6]. However, they, and later other workers, found that this resulted in suboptimal performance due

to significantly degraded energy resolution. The development and successful use of an improved, compact detector for this application was reported by Szypryt and colleagues [7], who provided an early report of the intra-operative use of a cadmium telluride detector. More recently, the excision of osteoid osteoma and successful follow-up in 12 patients has been reported [8] and Wioland and Sergent-Alaoui [9] have reviewed their experience of 175 radionuclide-guided excisions; both teams used scintillation detectors. Parathyroidectomy has been guided with the aid of a radiation probe, with resection of both ectopic parathyroid adenomas and hyperparathyroid tissue localised via their uptake of thallous-201 chloride [10] and more recently ^{99m}Tc-labelled sestamibi (MIBI) [11, 12].

Radiolabelled monoclonal antibodies may also be detected intra-operatively. The technique was first reported in 1984 by the group led by Martin, initially identifying occult tumour through detection of a polyclonal ^{131}I anti-CEA antibody in a patient with colorectal cancer [13]. The technique has been significantly refined since this time, using monoclonal antibodies with greater specificity and employing ^{125}I as the radiolabel [14–18]. The short range of the low-energy gamma rays emitted by ^{125}I precludes external imaging, but also acts to eliminate the detection of extraneous activity from distant sites of uptake. The 60-day half-life of ^{125}I also permits intra-operative detection after tumour to background activity levels have dropped to their optimum ratio, many days after administration of the radiolabelled antibody. Other groups have used this approach [19, 20] and the group of Di Carlo et al. have investigated pharmacological strategies for reducing the time delay necessary before operation [21]. With generally less success, radiolabelled

Table 1. Physical properties for radionuclides detected intra-operatively

Physical Property	Technetium-99m	Iodine-125	Iodine-123	Iodine-131	Indium-111	Fluorine-18	Thallium-201	Phosphorus-32
Half-life of radioactive decay	6.02 h	60.1 days	13.1 h	8.04 days	2.83 days	110 min	73.1 h	14.3 days
Energy of gamma ray emission	140 keV	27 keV	159 keV	364 keV	171, 247 keV	2@511 keV	68–80, 167 keV	None
Beta particle emission	None	None	None	606 keV (β_{max})	None	633 keV (β^+_{max})	None	1.71 MeV (β_{max})
Soft tissue thickness to reduce gamma rays to 50%	46 mm	17 mm	47 mm	63 mm	51 mm	71 mm (γ)	43 mm	8.2 mm (max. β^- range)
Thickness of lead to reduce gamma rays to 50%	0.17 mm	0.05 mm	0.5 mm	2.4 mm	0.9 mm	4.6 mm (γ)	0.06 mm	Not applicable
Thickness of lead to reduce gamma rays to 10%	0.9 mm	0.06 mm	1.2 mm	7.7 mm	2.5 mm	13.5 mm (γ)	0.9 mm	Not applicable

monoclonal antibodies (predominantly anti-CEA antibodies) optimised for external imaging by chelation to indium-111 have been evaluated intra-operatively, primarily for the investigation of colorectal cancer [22–26] and medullary thyroid cancer [27]. More recently monoclonal antibodies labelled with ^{99m}Tc have also been detected intra-operatively in ovarian cancer [28] and in colorectal carcinoma [29].

Neuroendocrine tumours expressing somatostatin receptors demonstrate uptake of radiolabelled forms of the somatostatin analogue octreotide [30] and have also been detected intra-operatively using these tracers. Both Wängberg [31] and Öhrvall and co-workers [32] have reported the successful use of ^{111}In-labelled DTPA-D-Phe^1-octreotide to detect a mixed group of predominantly abdominal cancers, and the same tracer has also been used to localise occult tumour in recurrent medullary thyroid carcinoma [33]. ^{125}I-Tyr^3-octreotide has been used by Schirmer et al. to identify gastroenteropancreatic tumours [34] and later by Martinez and colleagues to detect occult neuroblastoma [35]. Adams et al. have used both ^{111}In-labelled DTPA-D-Phe^1-octreotide and ^{99m}Tc (V)-dimercaptosuccinic acid (DMSA) to localise medullary thyroid carcinoma and gastroenteropancreatic tumours [36].

Metaiodobenzylguanidine (mIBG) has been developed as a tracer to target neural crest tumours [37] and has also been used intra-operatively in both ^{125}I- and ^{123}I-labelled forms to localise neuroblastoma, most notably in a recent series of 58 patients by Martelli and group [38].

Intra-operative Detector Design

To detect a sentinel node containing radiolabelled colloid both reliably and safely one requires a radiation detector designed for intra-operative use, and optimised for the application (Fig. 1). Using such a probe, the node must be detectable both transcutaneously and within the exposed surgical field by virtue of its radioactivity.

The system is required to perform reliably under surgical conditions, and the detector itself must demonstrate good stability over its expected lifetime. In considering the design features of such a probe, fundamental issues must be addressed relating to the physical performance of the detector; it is imperative that this is be at least adequate for the clinical application planned. Such aspects are discussed in the following sections. Equally important considerations of electromedical safety, including compliance with related legislative requirements, are also addressed, and a discussion of sterilisation techniques for the probe in surgical use is included in Chap. 7.

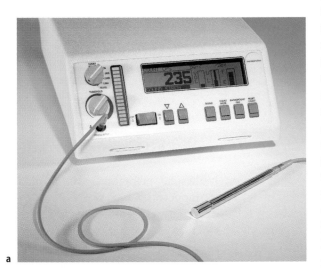

a

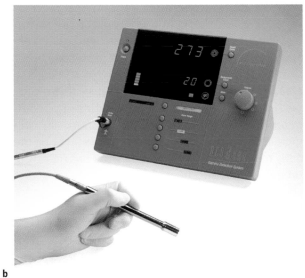

b

Fig. 1. a The Neoprobe 1500. **b** the Neo 2000. These two detector systems have been designed specifically for intra-operative sentinel node detection. Both use compact semiconductor radiation probes and have been developed by the same manufacturer. **Fig. b** illustrates recent progress in the design of the user interface (Courtesy of Neoprobe Corp.)

Aspects of the Sentinel Node Technique

In the sentinel node technique the detection task is somewhat different to the majority of clinical applications for intra-operative detection to date, and it is in general significantly more easily achieved. By definition the underlying concept is highly advantageous to the task, exploiting the exclusive transport of tracer through the lymphatic system to the first functioning lymph node. Distribution of tracer activity into the vascular structures of surrounding tissues is negligible, and the ratio of tracer uptake between the sentinel node and surrounding tissues is therefore extremely high; Kapteijn and colleagues found a mean percentage tracer uptake per gram tissue of 2.1 % in the sentinel node, versus 0.01 % for skin and 0.0035 % in subcutaneous fat [39]. Two recently published studies report that a sentinel node was demonstrated in 98 % [40] and 91 % [41] of patients investigated, and so the task becomes that of localising a radioactive sentinel node, or nodes, whose presence can be assumed with a high degree of confidence. Absolute levels of tracer uptake in the sentinel node are highly variable, but are consistent with easy detectability in the majority of locations and surroundings. Figure 2 illustrates the range of tracer activities recorded at our institution for a number of sentinel nodes removed at operation approximately 24 h after the tracer had been administered. Activity levels were determined in vitro immediately following resection using a calibrated gamma well counter, and are defined both in terms of the absolute activity level at the time of resection and as a percentage of the injected dose.

Spillover of tracer may occur due to use of colloids with smaller particle size, and this will certainly complicate the detection task through the presence of further radioactive lymph nodes. A more significant problem is caused when radioactivity is detected arising from the extensive residue of tracer retained in tissue at nearby injection site(s). The detrimental nature of this situation upon sentinel node detectability is discussed, together with strategies which may be adopted to minimise its effects.

Physical Principles Underlying Detector Performance

The radionuclide used to label all of the colloidal tracers employed in the detection of the sentinel

Fig. 2.
Tracer activity present within sentinel nodes at operation. Activity is recorded in-vitro using a calibrated gamma well counter immediately following resection of the nodes at biopsy, approximately 24 h after administration of tracer. Activity is defined both in terms of the absolute activity level at the time of operation and as a percentage of the injected dose

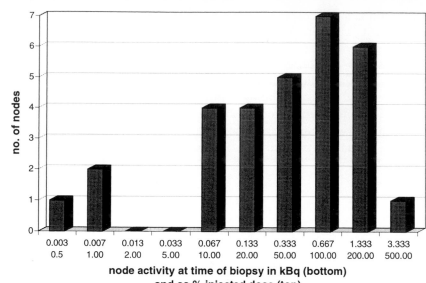

node is ^{99m}Tc. The physical characteristics of ^{99m}Tc are outlined here, and are listed in Table 1. These properties and their significance have also been reviewed by Thurston and colleagues for a number of radionuclides used intra-operatively [42].

Many factors will affect the detectability of the sentinel node. Both the absolute uptake of tracer activity within the node and the ratio of this activity to that of the surrounding tissue are critical to its detection. The size of the lymph node relative to the sensitive area of the detector face may also have an effect in that the probe may not be able to detect all activity present when it is distributed throughout a large node. It should, however, be noted that the uptake of colloidal tracer within a sentinel node is not always homogeneous; in fact a concentration of activity toward the afferent lymphatic ducts is often observed and should be taken into consideration when probing suspected sentinel nodes. This effect is particularly evident when the particle size of the colloid is relatively large.

The variability within the level of background activity is also highly relevant to detector performance [43] and its effect has been addressed in phantom studies performed by Hickernell et al. [44] and Hartsough [45]. This really only becomes a problem in the context of sentinel node detection when radioactivity from an injec-

tion site is located close to the area under investigation.

Fundamental physical principles also have a great effect upon the performance of the detector probe in localising sentinel nodes. The most significant of these factors is that of decreasing detection efficiency as the separation between the source and the detector face is increased. This geometrical effect is often termed the inverse-square law and refers to the physical relationship between the detected count rate and detector-source separation (d) for an idealised point source of activity and an infinitely small detector area, where the detected count rate will be proportional to $1/d^2$. The exact relationship is in practice modified at small separations by the increasing importance of the sensitive area of the detector face. Figure 3 illustrates the nature of the fundamental concept, and Fig. 4 details the exact count rate variation with increasing source-detector separation.

The count rate detected from a source of activity within the body will also decrease when the thickness of soft tissue interposed between it and the detector is increased. This is due to two effects: firstly gamma rays are absorbed by the intervening tissue, and additionally they are scattered, or deflected, out of the path of the detector as a result of its interaction with the tissue itself at an atomic level.

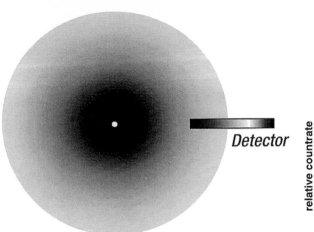

Fig. 3. Pictorial representation of the decrease in detected count rate (as grey shades) with increasing separation between a small volume source (white) and the detector

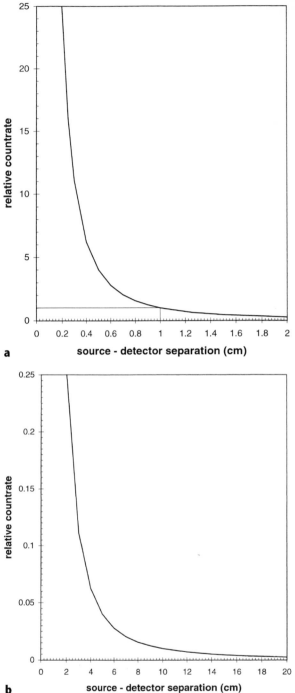

Fig. 4. Graphical representation of the relationship between detected count rate and source-detector separation from 0–2 cm (**a**) and from 0 to 20 cm (**b**)

The count rate detected from a source by a (collimated) detector is reduced with increasing thickness of an absorbing material such as soft tissue, due to a process termed attenuation, and the effect of attenuation is illustrated graphically in Fig. 5 for both ^{99m}Tc, and other radionuclides. The extent to which gamma rays are attenuated by tissue is heavily dependent upon the energy of the gamma ray but also varies with the extent to which both source and detector are collimated. Its effect is characterised by a fractional constant termed the linear attenuation coefficient μ, defined in cm^{-1}, and the exponential relationship that exists between the intensity of incident (I_0) and transmitted (I_x) gamma rays through a thickness (x) of absorbing tissue may be defined by the equation $I_0 = I_x\ e^{-\mu x}$. From this relationship the expected fraction of gamma rays transmitted through any thickness of intervening body tissue may be determined. At the 140-keV gamma energy of ^{99m}Tc the reduction in count rate due to the inverse-square effect arising from geometrical causes will predominate over the attenuating effect of soft tissue.

Scattering of radiation occurs due to a collision between the gamma ray and the outer electron of an atom (Fig. 6). The principal effects of this interaction (termed Compton scattering) in this context are that the incoming gamma ray loses some of its energy and is deflected from its path. Should the scattered gamma ray pass onward

Fig. 5.
Graphical representation of
the effect of tissue attenuation for
different radionuclides, characterised by the exponential relationship between detected count rate
and thickness of intervening
tissue

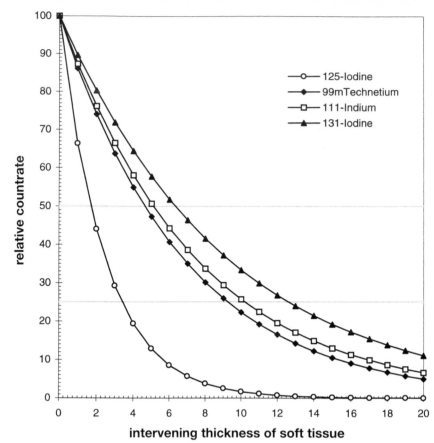

Fig. 6. Schematic representation of the scattering interaction
that takes place between an incoming gamma ray and the outer
shell electron of an atom lying within body tissue along its
path. The scattered gamma ray is deflected through an angle θ,
and loses some of its energy in the process

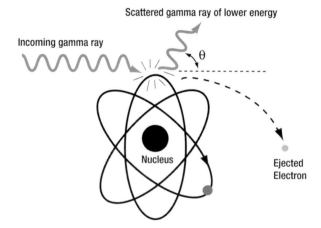

along its new path to the detector probe and be
accepted for detection, then it will appear to the
system as having originated from a site along this
line of travel and sufficient such events may be
erroneously represented as a false source of tracer
uptake. The loss of energy varies with the scattering angle, and scattering can occur at any angle.
The energy loss suffered by the gamma ray is at a
minimum for small angles of deflection, and it is
these gamma rays that are most likely to be accepted as valid events by the detector system. Scattering of an incoming gamma ray represents the
primary cause of events detected from a significant source of activity (e.g. injection site) sited
outside the direct zone of response of the detector, and its effects may be reduced under appropriate circumstances, but not eliminated, by
manipulating the range of gamma ray energies

(the energy "window") accepted for contribution to the detected signal. In practice, detection of both primary and scattered gamma rays from other sources may be reduced more significantly by the addition of collimation. These issues are discussed more fully below.

In summary, the effects of both attenuation by overlying tissue and the loss in counts due to geometrical causes (the inverse-square effect) may be minimised in practice if the thickness of this tissue can be reduced, either by re-positioning the region of the patient under investigation (as described by the displacement of overlying breast tissue when imaging) or by successively reducing the thickness of this overlying layer as a probe-guided resection of the node proceeds, leading to a resulting stepwise improvement in the detectability of the node with respect to transcutaneous measurements made before excision commences.

Detector Performance Characteristics

A number of design characteristics are important to the performance of the intra-operative detector. Detector sensitivity is critical, and may be defined here simply as the detected count rate per unit source activity (cps/MBq). Discussion of the optimal physical conditions under which detector sensitivity may be measured most meaningfully is somewhat more complex, and amongst other contributing factors the degree of detector collimation, the arrangement of source and detector, the source dimensions, the gamma ray energy acceptance window and the intervening media (tissue-equivalent scattering material or air) are all of real consequence to the validity and practical relevance of the result obtained.

Spatial resolution defines the ability of the detector to discriminate activity laterally, and is a key design consideration. Good spatial resolution may be inherent to the design of the detector (sometimes termed "integral collimation"), or may be achieved by use of a detachable collimator. The peak response of a detector at any depth will always lie along its central axis, and collimation acts to limit the acceptance of gamma rays striking the detector face from sources sited off the axis, the exact design properties of the collimator being chosen to manipulate the nature and extent of this fall-off in sensitivity with angle. Good spatial resolution is critical to achieving

adequate discrimination between the target radioactive structure under investigation, and any activity present within surrounding tissues – poor spatial resolution will increase the dimensions of the sensitive area beneath the probe face, leading to an apparent reduction in the relative tracer uptake, and lowering the recorded ratio between target and background count rates. Spatial resolution is conveniently characterised by defining the profile obtained when a detector is scanned laterally across the path of a point source of activity at a specified depth and with a specified medium intervening (either air or a tissue-equivalent scattering material such as water or perspex). The resulting profile should be symmetrical about the central axis of the detector, and is of the form of a Gaussian count distribution (Fig. 7). The width of the profile is a measure of the spatial resolution and may be defined as the full width at half the maximum height (FWHM) of the count profile, in units of distance. It can be demonstrated that the spatial resolution for any specific radionuclide, detector and source varies significantly with the degree of collimation, the depth of scattering media lying between source and detector, and the energy window chosen.

Detectors have the ability to discriminate between incoming gamma rays (e.g. between primary and scattered gamma radiation) by determining the energy deposited within the detector when the individual ray is absorbed. For the majority of detected events the full energy of the gamma ray is absorbed and recorded by the detector. The deposited energy is found from a knowledge of the physical properties of the detector material and associated components, and the precision with which this determination is performed is termed the energy resolution. Detector materials where the mechanism of detection is dominated by statistical variations in the efficiency with which each event is detected and processed, such as scintillation detectors, will give rise to an energy spectrum for detected gamma events whose main feature, termed a photopeak, resembles a Gaussian distribution similar to that illustrated in Fig. 7, and is centred about the actual energy of the incident gamma rays. When scattered radiation is present this will add a complex response pattern at energies lower than the photopeak, and this often contains a second,

Fig. 7.
Profile of the spatial response for a radiation detector to a point source of activity, and characterisation of spatial resolution as the full width of the profile at half its maximum height (FWHM)

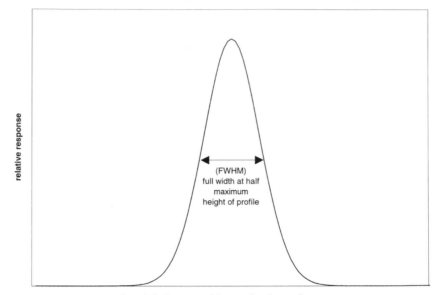

lateral displacement of detector face from point source

smaller peak which, though not totally separated, may be discerned from the main photopeak. The energy resolution of a detector may then be characterised as the percentage spread of the FWHM of the photopeak, in the same manner as for the quantification of spatial resolution. For other detector types such as semiconductor detectors, where the above statistical effects no longer dominate the characteristics of detection, this definition may not be applicable as the energy spectrum often contains significant inherent secondary features in addition to the primary photopeak. The measured energy resolution for any radiation detector is dependent upon the energy of the detected gamma ray, and accordingly will vary for different radionuclides. It is also strongly dependent upon the conditions of measurement, and in particular the presence of any intervening scattering medium which will act to introduce scattered radiation into the detected energy spectrum as described above. It is the energy resolution of a detector which defines its ability to reject scattered radiation originating from background activity by virtue of its lower energy, and the energy window (the region between the upper and lower energy acceptance threshold) may be determined for optimal detectability under any given circumstances.

The nature of the response field of a detector to a point source of activity may be understood when it is investigated within a tissue-equivalent scattering medium in three dimensions; both laterally about the axis of response, and at varying depths. This permits an appreciation of the lateral response of the detector at depth, and may be graphically expressed by means of an iso-response plot. An example of this is illustrated in Fig. 8, detailing the response of a detector probe without external collimation to a point source of ^{99m}Tc. An appreciation of the limiting response field of the detector assists when using the probe to survey wide areas, and to a lesser extent when probing at a later stage of the detection procedure in accordance with the "line-of-sight" technique detailed by Krag et al. [46]. This practical approach to intra-operative detection of the node is highly recommended and is discussed in more detail in Chap. 7.

Improved spatial resolution may be achieved by the use of collimation when it is a requirement for a specific application or individual situation. Collimation may be integral to the design of the detector probe shielding or may take the form of a removable additional component. The latter type comprises a forward directing "collar" of a heavily attenuating material such as steel or tungsten (tungsten having a better attenuation to weight ratio than lead) and should only be used when felt necessary, as it can add considerably to both the weight and dimensions of the probe

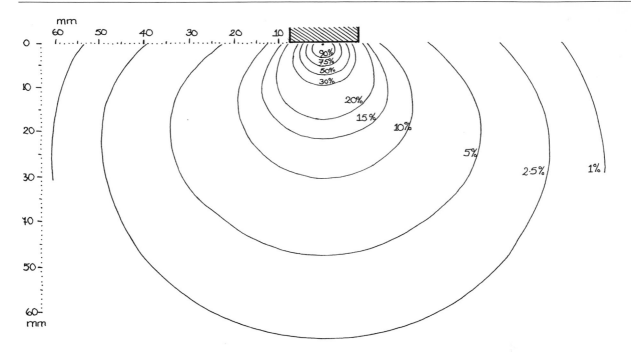

Fig. 8. Three-dimensional spatial response of a detection probe to a point source of ^{99m}-Tc. The detector has little internal collimation and so the response pattern is almost independent of angle; hence gamma rays originating from a site lying adjacent to the front surface of the probe will also be accepted. By adding a collimator the angle of acceptance for incoming gamma rays can be limited to a narrow range perpendicular to the detector face. The spatial response will then be modified, becoming much more directional and assuming a pattern similar to a "tear-drop" in overall form

and correspondingly reduces its manoeuverability and accessibility when performing an excisional sentinel node biopsy procedure. The collimator will reduce the exposed surface area of the sensitive zone at the detector face, thus reducing detector sensitivity – often considerably – and has an additional disadvantage in that the distance between the probe face and tissue is increased with a consequent significant loss in counting efficiency. However, the use of a collimator is strongly advised under appropriate conditions; it may render otherwise undetectable sentinel nodes lying close to significantly hotter sources of activity detectable through physically absorbing the scattered activity. This may be augmented in practice by the deliberate angulation of the detector probe away from known sites of extraneous tracer uptake. This strategy is discussed in more detail in Chap. 7,

and is both theoretically robust and very successful in practice.

The shielding of the detector probe housing with respect to gamma radiation incident upon its side face must also be adequate, and the need for this will vary with the radionuclide and clinical application. The key requirement here is that sufficient radiation from extraneous sources of activity be absorbed, such that the detection of hot sentinel nodes is not hampered by an artefactually increased count rate. An intermediate solution when moderately problematic neighbouring sources of activity are present is achieved by fitting a removable tungsten or steel secondary side-shield which acts to attenuate radiation impacting on the side face of the detector but does not reduce the surface area of the active detector face itself, thereby preserving the sensitivity of the detector as much as possible.

The key performance characteristics of any intra-operative radiation detector are to a great extent interdependent. Increase in spatial resolution may be gained at the expense of detector sensitivity, and a greater sensitivity may imply a loss in energy resolution. However, significant differences do still exist between the intrinsic performance of specific detector probes. Individual detector performance may be modelled for a given application by incorporating realistic biodistribution data into a computer model for the purpose of simulation studies, or in the construction of anthropomorphic physical phantoms. Often a combination of these two approaches is necessary for a full investigation to be performed [45, 47] such that optimum design characteristics and conditions for use may be identified.

Statistical Considerations Relating to Detection

The statistically reliable detection of suspicious radioactive structures is critical to the success of any intra-operative detection technique. This subject has been addressed previously [48, 49] and has been discussed in relation to the sentinel node detection task by Gulec and colleagues [50]. The Poisson statistics which characterise the random nature of the processes governing radioactive decay have been extensively detailed by Veall [51] and have also been addressed in respect of their application to signal detection criteria for scintigraphic image data [52].

A suitable criterion for statistical significance may be derived from these considerations, in relation to the difference between the count rate detected for the sentinel node (N) and for background (B). The variance of any single measured count is numerically equal to the recorded count itself, and the variance of the difference between these counts is defined as:

$$\text{variance } \sigma^2 = (N + B),$$

and hence:

$$\text{the standard deviation } \sigma = \sqrt{(N + B)}$$

If a threshold of three standard deviations, 3σ, is adopted as a criterion for the statistically significant detection of a sentinel node by virtue of its radioactivity, then there is greater than 99.7% chance that this is not due to the random error in detected counts alone. Thus, it is required that:

$$(N - B) \geq 3 \times \sqrt{(N + B)}.$$

If the mean of multiple counts are used then this criterion should be modified to the requirement that:

$$(\tilde{N} - \tilde{B}) \geq 3 \times \sqrt{(\tilde{N}/n + \tilde{B}/b)},$$

where $\tilde{N}$ is the mean node count and n the number of node counts performed, and $\tilde{B}$ is the mean background count and b the number of background counts performed. This has an important practical relevance in that use of a simple ratio between detected node and background counts, whilst a useful and conveniently determined aid to sentinel node detection, does not take account of the increasing statistical reliability gained when high recorded counts are obtained, either by use of longer counting times and multiple count samples, or by the use of a more sensitive detector probe. When the detection of a weakly active sentinel node is uncertain due to a limited increase only in the detected count rate on surveying, a recommended strategy is to record timed counts for at least 10–20 s, taken directly over the suspected node and over a representative background area. The statistical significance of the difference between these counts may then be at least estimated at this time as an aid to decision making.

Figure 9 illustrates the increasing statistical significance of 2:1, 4:1 and 8:1 node to background ratios as the recorded background count is increased due to increased counting time or greater detector sensitivity, and Fig. 10 demonstrates the decreased node to background ratio required to achieve a statistical significance of one, two and three standard deviations (σ) as the background count is increased.

Summary of Required Detector Characteristics

In conclusion, the inherent sensitivity of the detector is critically important to its overall performance in the intra-operative detection of sentinel nodes. Without good sensitivity, deeply situated sentinel nodes and sentinel nodes bearing low uptakes of tracer may not even be detectable. Equally importantly, good sensitivity must also be considered a prerequisite for the successful use of a detector probe when it is used with significant collimation to facilitate the detection of sentinel nodes sited near to sources of significant tracer activity. Collimation should be appropriate to the requirement, and should preferably be achieved by means of removable components for greater flexibility. The design of these should be consistent with good manoeuverability as far as is achievable given the necessary design con-

Fig. 9.
a The increasing statistical significance achieved by 2:1, 4:1 and 8:1 node to background ratios as the recorded background count is increased from 1 to 1000 (semilogarithmic plot). **b** The increasing statistical significance achieved by 2:1, 4:1 and 8:1 node to background ratios as the recorded background count is increased from 1 to 10 (linear plot)

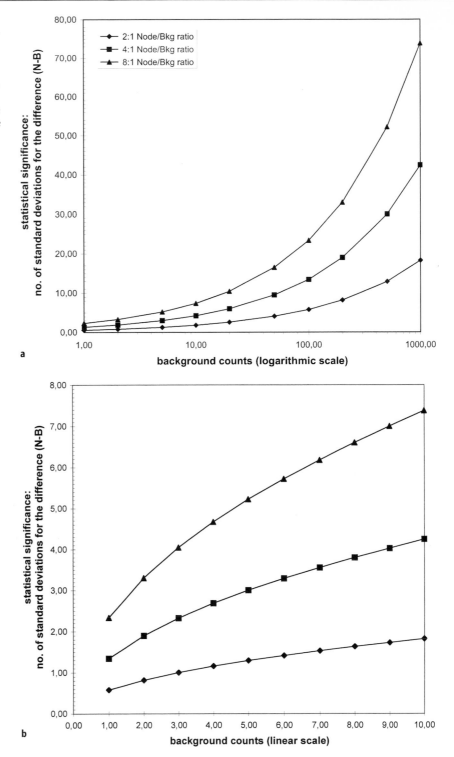

Fig. 10.
a The decreased node to background ratio required to achieve a statistical significance of one, two and three standard deviations (σ) as the background count is increased from 1 to 10 000 (semi-logarithmic plot). **b** The decreased node to background ratio required to achieve a statistical significance of one, two and three standard deviations (σ) as the background count is increased from 1 to 10 (linear plot)

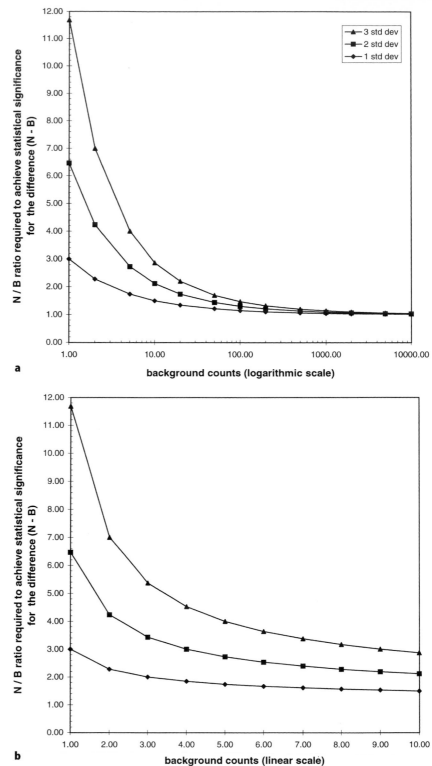

straints for shielding. Detector characteristics for the sentinel node technique have recently been evaluated for specific detector systems by Tiourina and colleagues [53] and Chap. 4 indicates a method by which the spatial resolution of detector probes may be conveniently assessed and ranked.

Intra-operative Detector Types

To date detectors used intra-operatively may be classified into two main groups: scintillation detectors and semiconductor detectors.

Scintillation Detectors

Scintillation detectors incorporate a material termed a scintillator as a means by which gamma radiation may be absorbed and detected. The detector itself is usually fabricated from a single crystal of the scintillation material, and the most commonly employed scintillators for intra-operative gamma ray detection are thallium-doped sodium iodide NaI(Tl) [44, 48] and caesium iodide CsI(Tl) [54]. The process of scintillation describes the interaction between the crystal structure of the detector and an incoming gamma ray when this impacts the crystal and its energy is absorbed by the detector as a result of the processes that then occur. These result in the generation of a minute burst of visible light energy within the crystal structure. This flash of light comprises typically a few thousand individual photons of light and is not perceptible to the human eye. It is detected and amplified by a photomultiplier tube, a specialised electronic device able to detect very low light intensities, and is converted into a measurable electronic pulse and amplified to a level suitable for further signal processing. The total light intensity generated is directly proportional to the absorbed gamma ray energy, although it fluctuates about a mean value due to the statistical processes underlying the generation and detection of the individual light photons. Hence energy discrimination is certainly possible with scintillation detectors, and provides a means by which scattered radiation may be rejected although the energy resolution for an intra-operative probe is relatively modest due to the spread in detected energies arising from the above-mentioned statistical uncertainties. The

processes of scintillation, detection, amplification and pulse processing all occur sufficiently rapidly to permit some tens of thousands of incident gamma rays per second to be accurately recorded. If a relatively thick scintillation crystal is used then the majority of incident gamma rays are detected and their energy is fully absorbed. Thus, scintillation detectors have good sensitivity for ^{99m}Tc.

Semiconductor Detectors

Semiconductor detectors use crystals of a semiconductor material, typically in the form of one or more small thin discs. Semiconductor detectors suitable for use at room temperatures include cadmium telluride (CdTe) [55–57] and more recently developed materials including cadmium zinc telluride (CdZnTe) [58] and mercuric iodide (HgI$_2$) [47, 59]. Cadmium telluride was the first semiconductor material to be used for intra-operative applications and has been widely employed [7, 60, 61] and cadmium zinc telluride has now been used clinically in commercial intra-operative detector systems [62]. Semiconductor detection materials for intra-operative use need a high atomic number to give a good stopping power for gamma rays, thus promoting efficient detection and a high sensitivity with respect to the dimensions of the detector, and high-purity crystals of useful dimensions can now be grown. Semiconductor detectors may be constructed to be extremely compact, and this has significantly benefited the design of probes for intra-operative use.

When an incident gamma ray is absorbed by a semiconductor detector, it interacts with the crystal by ionisation, leading to the production of a pair of charged particles having opposite electrical charge, termed an electron-hole pair. Typically 10–20 times as many of these charged particles are generated per unit gamma ray energy absorbed in a semiconductor crystal as visible light photons are released in a scintillator, and accordingly semiconductor detectors have the potential for very good energy resolution. When the semiconductor crystal is subjected to an electrical field by application of a bias voltage across its opposing faces, the charged particles, or charge carriers, may be detected at the electrodes, and the resulting current signal is amplified for further processing. In common with scintillation detectors, the energy detected is proportional to that deposited by the gamma ray. However, some of the charge carriers may be trapped at defect sites in the crystal and are not available for detection at the electrodes. This leads to a proportion of gamma ray events being recorded as having a lower energy, and the resulting energy spectrum will demonstate a plateau or tail located below the primary peak. This necessitates careful selection of the optimum energy window, as the events falling within the lower energy plateau are not necessarily due to scattered radiation, but may have arisen from gamma rays travelling directly in the path of the detector, whose energy has been incompletely recorded. This effect also limits the maximum crystal thickness across which the charge carriers can be successfully detected, and thereby reduces detector sensitivity for gamma rays of higher energy where the probability of their unhindered passage through the crystal is high. Strategies exist to minimise this effect, but typically the limiting energy for acceptable sensitivity of a semiconductor detector in clinical use is around 200–300 keV.

Ergonomic Considerations

Meaningful feedback of the instantaneous detected count rate is critical to the success of intra-operative detection techniques, and many workers have found an audio signal whose frequency or pulse rate rises with increasing count rate to be the optimum method for communicating variations in the detected signal to the surgeon when surveying wide areas for sites of tracer uptake. This has a clear advantage over a visual display of detected count rate in that the surgeon is not required to look away from the operative field while surveying the lymph node basin. Detected count rates may extend across many orders of magnitude and the audio signals described may be designed such that a single fixed relationship exists between count rate and audio frequency, leading to a relative insensitivity to subtle changes in count rate. Alternatively, the system may incorporate many sensitivity/count rate ranges, and selection of the optimal frequency range for audio feedback within the current count rate

range leads to greater auditory discrimination; however, this has a disadvantage in that it often requires the active involvement of a second person in the operating theatre.

Minor variations in the shape and design of the detector probe housing, and in the layout and nature of detector controls, are often a matter of personal preference. The readability of the display at a typical operating distance and the length of the cable between detector probe and control unit are other important ergonomic factors.

Practical Considerations

Quality Assurance

Quality assurance of the detector system will vary according to the exact device used, but optimal selection of energy windows is a requirement for most detectors. The best use of additional collimation will vary in accordance with the degree of collimation integral to the detector, and to the specific properties of the available removable collimators. A regular sensitivity test is highly recommended to guard against undetected gradual deterioration in performance over time. To facilitate this [129]I (gamma emissions at 29.7 and 33.6 keV, 15.7×10^6 year half-life) or [57]Co (122 kV gamma emission, half-life 267 days) standard sources may be purchased and conveniently used in a reproducible source-detector geometry. The practical implementation of this test is detailed in Chap. 7.

Electromedical Safety

By its nature an intra-operative radiation detector also comprises an item of electromedical equipment placed directly into the body cavity of a patient, and as such specific electromedical safety requirements must be satisfied to ensure its safe use in this regard. In common with other electrical equipment, the most significant single risk arises through the possibility of inducing ventricular fibrillation due to leakage current through the patient. This may arise from leakage originating within the device, or may be conducted via the device to earth due to an existing fault in another electrical device connected to the patient. Safe limits for leakage current and other electrical safety parameters have been defined under both normal and "single fault" conditions for medical electrical equipment by a safety standard produced by the International Electrotechnical Commission; IEC-60101 [63]. This document is internationally recognised and individual national standards are progressively harmonising with its requirements. Specific safety standards for intra-operative radiation detectors do not exist, but it is suggested that these devices meet the requirements for type CF devices, whose applied parts have the potential for direct electrical connection to the heart. The IEC document "Fundamental aspects of safety standards for medical electrical equipment" (IEC TR 60513 [64]) and the equivalent document published by the British Standards Institute (BSI PD 6573 [65]) are good sources for further information here.

Additionally, from April 1998 it has been a requirement within the European Union that all items of electromedical equipment possess CE Certification (popularly known as the "CE Mark") in accordance with the Medical Devices Directive (93/42/EEC) of the EU [66]. This does not specifically require that equipment be constructed to meet IEC 60101, but compliance with this standard is encouraged, and ensures that the requirements for electrical safety for CE Certification are met. In the United States the Food, Drugs and Cosmetics Act requires all electromedical equipment to be listed by and marketed in accordance with the Food and Drug Administration (FDA). As a minimum, the manufacturer is required to work within recommended quality systems and compliance with recognised electromedical safety standards is strongly advised, although not mandatory.

Prospective users are strongly advised to ensure that any intra-operative detector system considered for purchase meets all appropriate safety and legislative requirements.

The above regulations relate to the design and construction of a detection system, but do not by themselves guard against the existence of a fault in an individual piece of equipment. To ensure the continuing electrical safety of an intra-operative detector in regular use, it is important that an electrical safety test is performed upon acceptance and at least annually, supported by a thorough visual check for damage performed after each procedure. Specific attention should be paid to all electrical connections and particularly to the integrity of the probe cable, ensuring that its shielding is not damaged in any way. The detector itself should also be checked for visible damage. It must be stressed that equipment should never be used when damaged, as an electrical safety hazard may exist.

Finally, it should be noted that intra-operative detectors are susceptible to radiofrequency interference generated by electrocautery equipment. Spurious counts may be registered by the detector when electrocautery units are in use, and for this reason the two systems should never be used simultaneously. However, whilst this interference is not desirable in itself, experience suggests that the electromagnetic fields so generated are not likely to damage the detector system.

The Gamma Camera

Development of the Modern Gamma Camera

The gamma camera was devised by Hal Anger [67] in 1958. Although the design principles he first established still remain, in the 40 years since then a steady number of refinements have been introduced by many workers, dramatically improving its performance for clinical imaging.

Early cameras comprised a single circular detector with a gamma-ray sensitive field of view of approximately 300 mm diameter. Two-dimensional planar imaging only was possible and the images produced were output directly to film hard copy, in a process analogous to the generation of conventional X-ray films. In the early 1980s however, camera manufacturers integrated a computer system into the gamma camera which allowed the image data to be stored digitally for later processing and display. This development, together with improvements in the performance of the imaging detector itself, led to the development of the cross-sectional imaging technique single-photon emission tomography (SPET), analogous to X-ray computed tomography in the mode of its acquisition and processing of image data. Many nuclear medicine imaging procedures have developed in the intervening years to exploit this technique; particular examples include myocardial perfusion scintigraphy and functional

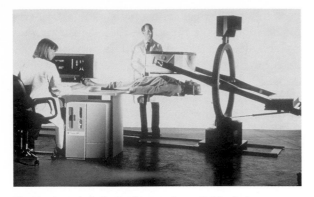

Fig. 11. A typical single detector large field of view gamma camera dating from the early 1990s (courtesy of GE Medical Systems)

neuroimaging. Further improvements in the performance of the detector itself, and advances in the capability of specifically designed gamma camera computer systems, have fostered more sophisticated strategies for acquiring and reviewing image data, and the development of a range of increasingly refined image processing techniques.

Contemporary gamma cameras now have rectangular detector heads, and these have a usable field of view of typically 400 mm × 500 mm (Fig. 11.). Reflecting a growth in the demand for nuclear medicine techniques, relatively recent commercial developments include the renaissance of gamma camera systems incorporating a second, or even third detector head (Fig. 12). Whilst increasing the overall cost, the clinical workload of multidetector systems is significantly

enhanced due to the increased efficiency with which both planar whole-body and SPET imaging studies may be performed when two or three detector heads simultaneously acquire image data.

For many clinically relevant applications, however, including that of the sentinel node imaging technique detailed in this book, it must be stressed that a single-headed planar gamma camera with its associated computer system remains sufficient to fulfil all technical requirements. The technique of sentinel node imaging is therefore clearly placed within the technical capability of every clinical nuclear medicine department.

Design Principles of the Gamma Camera

At the front face of the gamma camera lies a large, thin scintillation crystal. As described for scintillation detectors, a minute burst of visible light energy is generated within the crystal structure when it is impacted by an incoming gamma ray. It is for this reason that the Anger gamma camera is often referred to as a scintillation camera, and that nuclear medicine imaging is alternatively termed scintigraphy.

Figure 13 illustrates the operation of a contemporary digital gamma camera system. A hexagonal array of typically 50–70 discrete photomultiplier tubes are held in a fixed assembly at the back of the crystal, and when summed together their outputs record the pattern of light generated by the scintillation process. Signals from those photomultipliers registering a significant response to the detected gamma ray are processed by specialised hardware and software to determine the precise location of the gamma ray impact as x and y coordinates. These are then digitised and are directly stored to the computer to contribute to the formation of a scintigraphic image. As detailed for the scintillation detector, many tens of thousands of incident gamma rays per second may be accurately recorded. The acquired image is usually formed over a specified time interval, and consists of many individual detected gamma ray events whose overall pattern of distribution reflects the two-dimensional distribution of activity viewed by the detector.

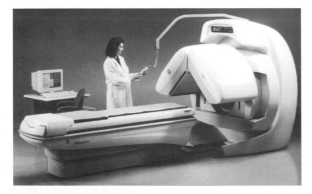

Fig. 12. A typical contemporay dual-detector large field of view gamma camera with variable detector geometry allowing differing detector orientations for SPET (courtesy of GE Medical Systems)

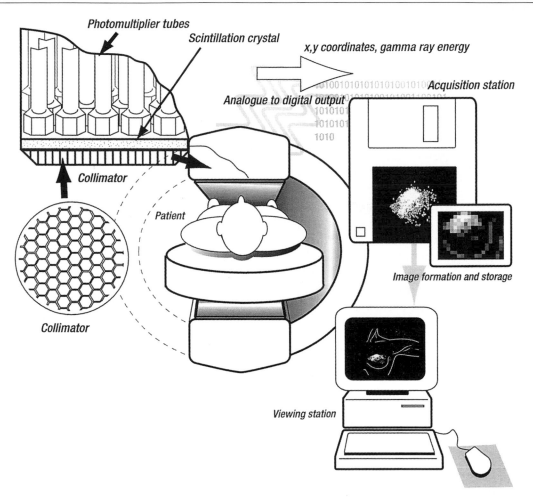

Photomultiplier tubes

Scintillation crystal

x,y coordinates, gamma ray energy

Acquisition station

Analogue to digital output

Collimator

Patient

Collimator

Image formation and storage

Viewing station

Fig. 13. Schematic representation of the operation of a digital gamma camera system. Gamma rays pass through the honeycomb structure of the collimator if travelling perpendicular to its face, and are detected within the scintillation crystal-photomultiplier tube assembly. The gamma ray energy and its location are determined by dedicated processing components. This information is then digitised and stored as a matrix of pixel counts in the data acquisition computer system. The resulting image may be displayed at a viewing station, after appropriate processing if required

The gamma ray energy absorbed by the crystal is also determined, enabling the rejection of scattered radiation. This process of energy selection is very similar to that used in intra-operative detectors, and is defined by means of a specified gamma ray energy window.

To generate a two-dimensional image of the relative distribution of tracer within the human body, the camera must include a means by which the angle of incoming gamma rays may be restricted – without this radiation from all locations will impact upon the entire face of the camera, as for a simple detector, and will blur the image detail contained beyond interpretation. This is achieved by means of a specialised collimator design, which may be likened in appearance to a lead plate mounted onto the front of the detector, comprising a finely detailed honeycomb-like structure, uniformly perforated by many tens of thousands of regularly spaced hexagonal holes separated by thin walls or septa. These form a physical barrier to those gamma rays arriving other than effectively perpendicular to the front face of the detector. The absorptive property of the lead collimator represents the single most significant cause for the relatively low detector sensitivity of the gamma camera, and in specifying its properties a design trade-off exists between this sensitivity (defined by the detected count rate per unit source activity) and the fineness of image detail (spatial resolution) that is ultimately achievable under optimal imaging conditions. Each gamma camera utilises a range of collimators individually designed to optimise either detector sensitivity or spatial resolution by varying degrees, and constructed to be interchangeable components of the detector.

The gamma camera computer is usually integral to the camera system and provides an interface through which the acquisition of digital image data may be controlled by the operator. Image data are stored as a two-dimensional pixel matrix of detected gamma events, and may be collected in a number of formats, e.g. as a single-frame "static" projection or as a continuous dynamic sequence of short time frames at a specified projection. Whole-body scans may be generated by moving the integrated patient couch with respect to the detector(s) at a specified constant speed along the length of the patient, whilst acquiring a single, scanned view of the distribution of tracer throughout the body. Whole- or part-body scanned images are useful in interpreting lymphatic drainage from melanomas, particularly of the lower limb.

Review of a sequence of dynamic frames in cine form allows the underlying time dependency of tracer uptake to be clearly visualised for the structures imaged. Additionally, specific individual images may be added together, subtracted from each other and otherwise manipulated for optimal display. It is possible to obtain sentinel node images with very high resolution, as the tracer activity is often superficially located with minimal overlying tissue. This may be exploited by using a high-resolution collimator, a fine digitisation matrix (optimally 256 × 256) and careful patient positioning – always minimising distance between the source of activity and the detector face. Through these strategies individual lymphatic ducts and their interrelationship are made visible, and detection of sentinel nodes lying very close to the injection site is enhanced.

References

1. Selverstone B, Sweet WH, Robinson CV. The clinical use of radioactive phosphorus in the surgery of brain tumours. *Ann Surg* 1949; 130:643–651

2. Harris CC, Bigelow RR, Francis JE, Kelly GG, Bell P. A CsI(Tl) crystal surgical scintillation probe. *Nucleonics* 1956; 14:102–108

3. Morris AC, Barclay TR, Tanida R, Nemcek JV. A miniaturised probe for detecting radioactivity at thyroid surgery. *Phys Med Biol* 1971; 16:397–404

4. Lennquist S, Persliden J, Smeds S. Intraoperative scintigraphy in surgical treatment of thyroid carcinoma: evaluation of a new technique. *World J Surg* 1986; 10:711–717

5. Lennquist S, Persliden J, Smeds S. The value of intraoperative scintigraphy as a routine procedure in thyroid carcinoma. *World J Surg* 1988; 12:586–592

6. Harvey WC, Lancaster JL. Technical and clinical characteristics of a surgical biopsy probe. *J Nucl Med* 1981; 22:184–186

7. Szypryt EP, Hardy JG, Colton CL. An improved technique of intra-operative bone scanning. *J Bone Joint Surg [Br]* 1986; 68:643–646

8. Kirchner B, Hillmann A, Lottes G, Sciuk J, Bartenstein P, Winkelmann W, Schober O. Intraoperative, probe-guided curettage of osteoid osteoma. *Eur J Nucl Med* 1993; 20:609–613

9. Wioland M, Sergent-Alaoui A. Didactic review of 175 radionuclide-guided excisions of osteoid osteoma. *Eur J Nucl Med* 1996; 23:1003–1011

10. Ubhi CS, Hardy JG, Pegg CAS. Mediastinal parathyroid adenoma: a new method of localization. *Br J Surg* 1984; 71:859–860

11. Martinez DA, King DR, Romshe C, Lozano RA, Morris JD, O'Dorisio MS, Martin E. Intraoperative identification of parathyroid gland pathology: a new approach. *J Pediatr Surg* 1995; 30:1306–1309

12. Bonjer HJ, Bruining HA, Pols HAP, de Herder WW, van Eijck, Breeman WAP, Krenning EP. Intraoperative nuclear guidance in benign hyperparathyroidism and parathyroid cancer. *Eur J Nucl Med* 1997; 24:246–251

13. Aitken DR, Hinkle GH, Thurston MO, Tuttle SE, Martin DT, Olsen J, Haagensen DE, Houchens D, Martin EW. A gamma-detecting probe for radioimmune detection of CEA-producing tumors: successful experimental use and clinical case report. *Dis Colon Rectum* 1984; 27:279–282

14. Arnold MW, Schneebaum S, Berens A, Petty L, Mojzisik C, Hinkle G, Martin EW. Intraoperative detection of colorectal cancer with radioimmunoguided surgery and CC49, a second-generation monoclonal antibody. *Ann Surg* 1992; 216:627–632

15. Arnold MW, Schneebaum S, Berens A, Mojzisik C, Hinkle G, Martin EW. Radioimmunoguided surgery challenges traditional decision making in patients with primary colorectal cancer. *Surgery* 1992; 112:624–630

16. Burak WE, Schneebaum S. Radioimmunoguided surgery: recurrent clinical trials and applications. *Semin Col Rectal Surg* 1995; 6:225–233

17. Burak WE, Schneebaum S, Kim JA, Arnold MW, Hinkle G, Berens A, Mojzisik C, Martin EW. Pilot study evaluating the intraoperative localisation of radiolabelled monoclonal antibody CC83 in patients with metastatic colorectal carcinoma. *Surgery* 1995; 118:103–108

18. Arnold MW, Hitchcock CL, Young DC, Burak WE, Bertsch DJ, Martin EW. Intra-abdominal patterns of disease dissemination in colorectal cancer identified using radioimmunoguided surgery. *Dis Colon Rectum* 1996; 39:509–513

19. Dawson PM, Blair SD, Begent RHJ, Kelly AMB, Boxer GM, Theodorou NA. The value of radioimmunoguided surgery in first and second look laparotomy for colorectal cancer. *Dis Colon Rectum* 1991; 34:217–222

20. Di Carlo V, Badellino F, Stella M, De Nardi P, Fazio F, Percivale P, Bertoglio S, Schenone F, Benevento A, Carcano G, Dominioni L, Dionigi R. Role of B72.3 iodine-125-labeled monoclonal antibody in colorectal cancer detection by radioimmunoguided surgery. *Surgery* 1994; 115:190–198

21. Stella M, De Nardi P, Paganelli G, Magnani P, Mangili F, Sassi I, Baratti D, Gini P, Zito F, Cristallo M, Fazio F, Di Carlo V. Avidin-biotin system in radioimmunoguided surgery for colorectal cancer: advantages and limits. *Dis Colon Rectum* 1994; 37:335–343

22. Curtet C, Vuillez JP, Daniel G, Aillet G, Chetanneau, Visset J, Kremer M, Thédrez P, Chatal JF. Feasibility study of radioimmunoguided surgery of colorectal carcinomas using indium-111-CEA-specific monoclonal antibody. *Eur J Nucl Med* 1990; 17:299–304

23. Davidson BR, Waddington WA, Short MD, Boulos PB. Intraoperative localization of colorectal cancers using radiolabelled monoclonal antibodies. *Br J Surg* 1991; 78:664–670

24. Kuhn JA, Corbisiero RM, Buras RR, Carroll RG, Wagman LD, Wilson LA, Yamauchi D, Smith MM, Kondo R, Beatty JD. Intraoperative gamma detection probe with presurgical antibody imaging in colon cancer. *Arch Surg* 1991; 126:1398–1403

25. Reuter M, Montz R, de Heer K, Schäfer H, Klapdor R, Desler K, Schreiber HW. Detection of colorectal carcinomas by intaoperative RIS in addition to preoperative RIS: surgical and immunohistochemical findings. *Eur J Nucl Med* 1992; 19:102–109

26. Abdel Nabi H, Doerr RJ, Balu D, Rogan L, Farrell EL, Evans NH. Gamma probe assisted ex vivo detection of small lymph node metastases following the administration of indium-111-labelled monoclonal antibodies to colorectal cancers. *J Nucl Med* 1993; 34:1818–1822

27. Peltier P, Curtet C, Chatal JF, Le Doussal JM, Daniel G, Aillet G, Gruaz-Guyon, Barbet J, Delange M. Radio-immunodetection of medullary thyroid cancer using a bispecific anti-CEA/anti-indium-DTPA antibody and an indium-111-labeled DTPA dimer. *J Nucl Med* 1993; 34:1267–1273

28. Ind TEJ, Granowska M, Britton KE, Morris G, Lowe DG, Hudson CN, Shepherd JH. Peroperative radioimmunodetection of ovarian carcinoma using a hand-held gamma detection probe. *Br J Cancer* 1994; 70:1263–1266

29. Moffat FL, Vargas-Cuba RD, Serafini AN, Jabir AM, Sfakianakis GN, Sittler SY, Robinson DS, Crichton VZ, Subramanian R, Murray JH, Klein JL, Hanna MG, DeJager RL. Preoperative scintigraphy and operative probe scintimetry of colorectal carcinoma using technetium-99m-88BV59. *J Nucl Med* 1995; 36:738–745

30. Krenning EP, Kwekkeboom DJ, Bakker WH, Breeman WAP, Kooij PPM, Oei HY, van Hagen M, Postema PTE, deJong M, Reubi JC, Visser TJ, Reijs AEM, Hofland LJ, Koper JW, Lamberts SWJ. Somatostatin receptor scintigraphy with [111-In-DTPA-D-Phe¹] and [123-I-Tyr³]-octreotide: the Rotterdam experience with more than 1000 patients. *Eur J Nucl Med* 1993; 20:716–731

31. Wängberg B, Forssell-Aronsson E, Tisell LE, Nilsson O, Fjälling M, Ahlman H. Intraoperative detection of somatostatin-receptor-positive neuroendocrine tumours using indium-111-labelled DTPA-D-Phe¹-octreotide. *Br J Cancer* 1996; 73:770–775

32. Öhrvall U, Westlin JE, Nilsson S, Juhlin C, Rastad J, Lundqvist H, Åkerström G. Intraoperative gamma detection reveals abdominal endocrine tumors more efficiently than somatostatin receptor scintigraphy. *Cancer* 1997; 80:2490–2494

33. Waddington WA, Kettle AG, Heddle RM, Coakley AJ. Intraoperative localization of recurrent medullary carcinoma of the thyroid using indium-111 pentreotide and a nuclear surgical probe. *Eur J Nucl Med* 1994; 21: 363–364

34. Schirmer WJ, O'Dorisio TM, Schirmer TP, Mojzisik CM, Hinkle GH, Martin EW. Intraoperative localization of neuroendocrine tumors with 125-I-TYR(3)-octreotide and a hand-held gamma detecting probe. *Surgery* 1993; 114:745–752

35. Martinez DA, O'Dorisio MS, O'Dorisio TM, Qualman SJ, Caniano DA, Teich S, Besner GE, King DR. Intraoperative detection and resection of occult neuroblastoma: a technique exploiting somatostatin-receptor expression. *J Pediatr Surg* 1995; 30:1580–1589

36. Adams S, Baum R, Hertel A, Wenisch HJC, Staib-Sebler E, Herrmann G, Encke A, Hör G. Intraoperative gamma probe detection of neuroendocrine tumors. *J Nucl Med* 1998; 39:1155–1160

37. Hoefnagel CA. Metaiodobenzylguanidine and somatostatin in oncology: role in the management of neural crest tumours. *Eur J Nucl Med* 1994; 21:561–581

38. Martelli H, Ricard M, Larroquet M, Wioland M, Paraf F, Fabre M, Josset P, Helardot PG, Gauthier F, Terrier-Lacombe M-J, Michon J, Hartmann O, Tabone MD, Patte C, Lumbroso J, Grüner J (1998) Intraoperative localization of neuroblastoma in children with 123-I or 125-I radiolabeled metaiodobenzylguanidine. *Surgery* 123: 51–57

39. Kapteijn BAE, Nieweg OE, Muller SH, Liem IH, Hoefnagel CA, Rutgers EJT, Kroon BBR. Validation of gamma probe detection of the sentinel node in melanoma. *J Nucl Med* 1997; 38:362–366

40. Veronesi U, Paganelli G, Galimberti V, Viale G, Zurrida S, Bedoni M, Costa A, deCicco C, Geraghty JG, Luini A, Sacchini V, Veronesi P. Sentinel node biopsy to avoid axilliary dissection in breast cancer with clinically negative lymph nodes. *Lancet* 1997; 349:1864–1867

41. Krag D, Weaver D, Ashikaga T, Moffat F, Klimberg VS, Shriver C, Feldman S, Kusminsky R, Gadd M, Kuhn J, Harlow S, Beitsch P. The sentinel node in breast cancer – a multicenter validation study. *N Engl J Med* 1998; 339: 941–946

42. Thurston MO, Kaehr JW, Martin EW III, Martin EW jr. Radionuclide of choice for use with an intraoperative probe. *Antibody Immunoconj Radiopharm* 1991; 4:595–601

43. Woolfenden JM, Barber HB. Radiation detector probes for tumor localisation using tumor-seeking radioactive tracers. *AJR* 1989; 153:35–39

44. Hickernell TS, Barber HB, Barrett HH, Woolfenden JM. Dual-detector probe for surgical tumor staging. *J Nucl Med* 1988; 1101–1106

45. Hartsough NE, Barrett HH, Barber HB, Woolfenden JM. Introperative tumor detection: relative performance of single-element, dual-element, and imaging probes with

various collimators. *IEEE Trans Med Imag* 1995; 14: 259–265

46. Krag DN, Ashikaga T, Harlow SP, Weaver DL. Development of sentinel node targeting technique in breast cancer patients. *Breast J* 1998; 4:67–74

47. Kwo DP, Barber HB, Barrett HH, Hickernell TS, Woolfenden JM. Comparison of NaI(Tl), CdTe, and HgI₂ surgical probes: effect of scatter compensation on probe performance. *Med Phys* 1991; 18:382–389

48. Barber HB, Barrett HH, Woolfenden JM, Myers KJ, Hickernell TS. Comparison of in vivo scintillation probes and gamma cameras for detection of small, deep tumors. *Phys Med Biol* 1989; 34:727–739

49. Waddington WA, Davidson BR, Todd-Pokropek A, Boulos PB, Short MD. Evaluation of a technique for the intraoperative detection of a radiolabelled monoclonal antibody against colorectal cancer. *Eur J Nucl Med* 1991; 18: 964–972

50. Gulec SA, Moffat FL, Carroll RG, Krag DN. Gamma probe guided sentinel node biopsy in breast cancer. *Q J Nucl Med* 1997; 41:251–261

51. Veall N (1971) Statistical factors affecting radioactivity measurements. In: Belcher EH, Vetter H (eds) *Radioisotopes in medical diagnosis*. London: Butterworths

52. Evans AL (1981) The quest for a "figure of merit". In: *The evaluation of medical images*. Adam Hilger, Bristol

53. Tiourina T, Arends B, Huysmans D, Rutten H, Lemaire B, Muller S. Evaluation of surgical gamma probes for radioguided sentinel node localisation. *Eur J Nucl Med* 1998; 25:1224–1231

54. Wilson LA, Kuhn JA, Corbisiero RM, Smith M, Beatty JD, Williams LE, Rusnak M, Kondo RL, Demidecki AJ. A technical analysis of an intraoperative radiation detection probe. *Med Phys* 1992; 19:1219–1223

55. Scheiber C, Chambron J. CdTe detectors in medicine: a review of current applications and future perspectives. *Nucl Instrum Methods* 1992; A322:604–614

56. Eisen Y. Current state-of-the-art applications utilizing CdTe detectors. *Nucl Instr Meth* 1992; A322:596–603

57. Squillante MR, Entine G. New applications of CdTe nuclear detectors. *Nucl Instr Meth* 1992; A322:569–574

58. Barber HB. Application of II-VI materials to nuclear medicine. *J Electronic Materials* 1996; 25:1232–1240

59. Barber HB, Barrett HB, Hickernell TS, Kwo DP, Woolfenden JM, Entine G, Ortale Baccash C. Comparison of NaI(Tl), CdTe, and HgI₂ surgical probes: physical characterization. *Med Phys* 1991; 18:373–381

60. Hinkle GH, Abdel-Nabi H, Miller EA, Schlanger LE, Houchens DP, Thurston MO, Aitken DR, Mojzisik CM, Olsen JO, Tuttle SE, Hansen HJ, Haagensen DE, Martin EW. Radioimmunodetection of implanted tumors with gamma probe. *NCI Monogr* 1987; 3:83–87

61. Roncari G, Benevento A, Bianchi L, Ceriani L, Garancini S, Lovisolo J, Dionigi R. Performance evaluation of a hand-held gamma probe used for radioimmunoguided surgery. *J Nucl Biol Med* 1993; 37:21–25

62. Cox CE, Pendas S, Cox JM, Joseph E, Shons AR, Yeatman T, Ku NN, Lyman GH, Berman C, Haddad F, Reintgen DS. Guidelines for sentinel node biopsy and lymphatic mapping of patients with breast cancer. *Ann Surg* 1998; 227:645–653

63. International Electrotechnical Commission. Medical Electrical Equipment – Part 1: General requirements for safety. IEC 60101-1 (1988-12). Geneva: IEC, 1988

64. International Electrotechnical Commission. Fundamental aspects of safety standards for medical electrical equipment. IEC TR 60513 (1994–01). Geneva: IEC, 1994

65. British Standards Institute. Fundamental aspects of safety standards for medical electrical equipment. BS PD 6573. London: BSI, 1994

66. Medical Devices Directive 93/42/EEC. Official Journal of the European Communities N° L189/90. (ISBN 0-119-1221-38)

67. Anger HO. Scintillation camera. *Rev Sci Instrum* 1958; 29:27–33

Further Reading

The interested reader is referred to the following books. These are excellent texts for further information regarding the physical principles underlying radiation dectection. The first is aimed at a general readership; the second is a more comprehensive physics text.

Sorenson JA, Phelps ME. *Physics in nuclear medicine.* 2nd edn. Orlando: Grune and Stratton, 1987. (ISBN 0-8089-1804-4)

Knoll GF. *Radiation detection and measurement, 2nd edn.* New York: John Wiley, 1989. (ISBN 0-471-81504-7)

CHAPTER 4

How To Choose a Probe *

ALLEN J. BRITTEN

Introduction

Intra-operative gamma probes are increasingly used to localise the first draining lymph node from a tumour, the sentinel node, in melanoma and breast cancer [1–5]. A wide range of probe systems are available with different detector materials, detector sizes and collimation, and evaluation is required prior to purchase and use. The basic physical probe performance can be described by the spatial resolution, sensitivity and count rate linearity [6]. Comparison of these parameters allows us to rank different systems in terms of relative performance for each parameter, but give us little insight into relative performance in localising sentinel nodes. For example, which probe is superior if one has a spatial resolution 5.6 mm better than the other but a 20% poorer sensitivity? This paper describes, validates and applies a methodology to allow comparison of probe performance in practical terms related to the task of sentinel node localisation in melanoma and breast cancer. The basis of the approach is that the response of a probe to multiple sources, such as the injection site and sentinel node, can be calculated by suitable shifting, scaling and addition of the probe's sensitivity profiles at the appropriate source depths. Measurements are made of the sensitivity of the probe from its response to a technetium-99m point source at different depths in water, with the source moved off-axis to produce curves referred to as sensitivity profiles, in cps/MBq at varying distances from the probe axis. The response of the detector to multiple sources can be simply estimated by adding several sensitivity profiles, with appropriate shifts along the abscissa to simulate the separation between the

sources, and scaling to reflect different amounts of activity in each source. The power of simulation is that we can easily investigate different separations between the injection site and node, different absolute activities in the injection site and node, and different ratios of activity in the two areas. We can also simulate multiple injection sites, as commonly used in clinical practice. Previously workers in other applications of intra-operative gamma probes have carried out extensive measurements with specific phantoms and sources [7], but this approach involves a prohibitive number of measurements when comparing multiple source locations, different activity ratios between injection site and node, and several probes.

This paper reports the application of this method for the evaluation of five probes, ranking them in terms directly related to their ability to localise lymph nodes in the presence of scatter background from the injection site. A very wide range of node and injection site relative positions and activities are met in clinical practice and, though the methodology presented can be used to simulate all of these situations, the main aim of this work is to compare probe performance in the same physical situation. In this context we have chosen the physical conditions such that the probe performance is tested to its limits, rather than attempt to model the full range of conditions met in clinical practice.

Materials and Methods

Probes

Measurements were made with the Neoprobe 1500 (Neoprobe Corporation, Dublin, Ohio, USA) and Europrobe (Eurorad, Sevres, France) systems, each

* First published in *Eur J Nucl Med* 26, 1999.

with two probes, and one probe with the Navigator GGS system (United States Surgical Corporation, Norwalk, Conn., USA). The Neoprobe 1500 system had cadmium-zinc-telluride probes of 19 mm and 14 mm diameter used with removeable collimators fitted; these are referred to as N19 and N14 respectively. The Europrobe had a 16-mm CsI (Tl) detector (ECSI), and an 11-mm CdTe probe (ECDT), with only internal collimation. A 14-mm CdTe probe with internal collimation was used on the Navigator GGS system (NAV). All sizes are nominal outside diameters of the probes before added collimation. The lower energy threshold on the N19 probe was set to 145 (arbitrary units) and some measurements were repeated at 150 to illustrate how the method can be applied to performance optimisation. The N14 probe lower energy threshold was set to 150; the upper energy threshold was set to 255 for both Neoprobe probes. The Europrobes were operated with an energy window of 110–170 keV, and the Navigator was tested with a 95 keV lower energy threshold.

Basic Performance Measurements

Sensitivity profiles were obtained with a fixed source at depth in water, and the probe moved laterally. The source was formed by a drop of ^{99m}Tc filling a 2-mm-diameter hole 3 mm deep in a 5-mm-thick, 20-mm-square perspex block, sealed with adhesive tape. All source activities were measured in the same radioisotope calibrator, with a daily variation around 2% and error in the absolute activity of less than 10%. The source block was positioned at 50 mm depth in a water bath, 250 mm long by 150 mm wide by 150 mm water depth. A frame with a clamp held the probe perpendicular to the water surface, with an estimated positioning error of ± 0.5 mm. Measurements were made at source centre-to-probe depths (D) in water of 5 mm, 10 mm, 20 mm, 30 mm and 50 mm, obtained by moving the probe tip beneath the water surface. Paired count rates were measured with the probe tip submerged 20 mm in water and not submerged, with a fixed source depth D of 30 mm, to check that possible increased multiple scatter with the tip submerged was negligible.

Sensitivity profiles in cps/MBq were obtained over the lateral range – 60 mm to + 120 mm from the source centre. Counts were taken at 2.5-mm intervals at up to ± 20 mm off-axis, then at ± 25 mm and at each 10-mm interval up to – 60 mm and + 120 mm. The central part of the profile was recorded with a source activity of 0.6–1 MBq, with the source increased up to a maximum of 23 MBq for points at more than 40 mm off-axis in order to achieve more than 500 counts within 60 s counting time.

Data were entered onto a computer spreadsheet (Microsoft Excel V7.0), decay corrected, linearly interpolated to 2.5-mm intervals and expressed as cps/MBq. Linear interpolation for points beyond 30 mm off-axis introduced a maximum error of 6% in the interpolated points in the region of maximum curvature of the profiles. Basic performance measures were recorded as the sensitivity on-axis (cps/MBq), and the full-width at half-maximum (FWHM) of the sensitivity profiles, at 5 mm, 10 mm, 20 mm, 30 mm and 50 mm water depths.

Validation of the simulation was performed with three probes (N19, ECSI, ECDT) by measuring the sensitivity profiles from two ^{99m}Tc sources in water, one at 5 mm depth representing the injection site, and one at 30 mm depth representing the node. The ratio of node-to-injection site activity (NIR) was 1:60. The measured sensitivity profiles were compared with the simulated data for this configuration.

Simulations

Simulation involves modelling an idealised form of the clinical situation (Fig. 1), with flat skin surface and the probe perpendicular to the skin surface. Multiple injection sites are frequently used, either around a tumour or the melanoma skin surface scar [1]. For simulations relevant to melanoma a dual injection was modelled as two equal activity injections, 20 mm apart and 5 mm deep, with the node-to-injection site (NS) distance and the probe-to-injection distance (PID) defined from the injection site nearest to the node (Fig. 1). Multiple injections could be modelled in the breast simulations, but with wide variability dependent upon each patient it would be hard to select a representative peritumoral injection geometry, so a tumour centre single injection at 30 mm depth was simulated.

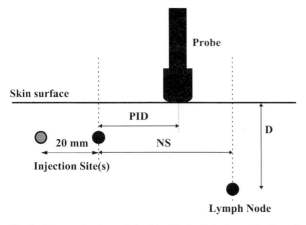

Fig. 1. Schematic view of the idealised clinical positioning of injection site, node and probe, all lying in the same vertical plane. For simulations with two injections at 20 mm separation (dual injection), the probe-to-injection site distance (*PID*) is from the closest injection site

Simulations were performed with a node depth of 30 mm for all probes, with further simulations carried out for the N19 probe at node depths of 10 mm, 20 mm and 50 mm, and a 5-mm-deep-dual injection.

Simulations were performed for NIRs of 1:50, 1:100 and 1:200. This range was chosen since preliminary investigation showed that the limiting performance of the probes was reached within this NIR range, for identification of nodes within 110 mm of the injection site. Simulations were carried out with injection site activities (ISA) of 1 MBq, 2.5 MBq and 10 MBq.

To illustrate the simulation procedure, consider the case of a 5-mm-deep injection with a 20-mm-deep lymph node at 50 mm separation (NS) from the injection, with NIR 1:50. The injection site is represented by the 5-mm-deep sensitivity profile, whilst the 20-mm-deep sensitivity profile representing the node response is shifted by 50 mm in the positive off-axis direction, multiplied by 1/50 and added to the injection site sensitivity profile. The simulated counts profile therefore represents the detected count rate, per MBq in the injection site, which the probe would register if travelling along the skin surface on a line drawn between the injection site and node positions. This is the optimal line of approach for the probe to identify two sources.

The simulations were repeated for NS distances from 30 mm to 110 mm in 5-mm steps, so that a series of simulated profiles are produced corresponding to increasing node distance from the injection site.

Analysis of Simulated Data

The aim of the analysis is to determine the minimum separation between injection site and node which is required to allow identification of the node. The simulated count response values are visually inspected to identify a peak *P* cps/MBq followed by a minimum *M* cps/MBq before the probe reaches the main injection site peak (Fig. 2). The percentage peak reduction (PPR) from the node peak to minimum is defined as $(P-M)/P \times 100\%$, and the graph of PPR versus NS indicates when a node may be identified (Fig. 3a). Based upon laboratory experience with the probes a detection threshold PPR of 25% was set. The minimum NS at which PPR is 25% is referred to as MNS [25%]. There must also be sufficient counts to allow confident identification of a fall in counts from *P* to *M*, and a three standard deviation drop from the node peak *P* to the following minima is set as a detection criterion. The ratio of $(P-M)$ to the standard deviation of $(P-M)$ is the number of standard deviations in the difference between peak *P* and dip *M*, referred to as $No.\ No$ was simply calculated from the Poisson statistics of the final

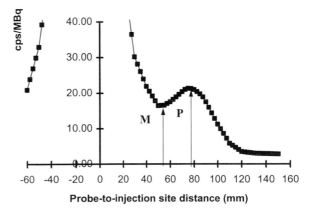

Fig. 2. Example of simulation data for N19 probe with NIR 1:50, injection depth 5 mm, node depth 30 mm, dual injection and 80 mm separation between node and injection sites. The curve is scaled so that the low count rate peak from the node can be seen. Note that the count rate at the injection site is 185 times higher than the count rate at the node. The peak node counts *P* and minimum counts *M* are shown

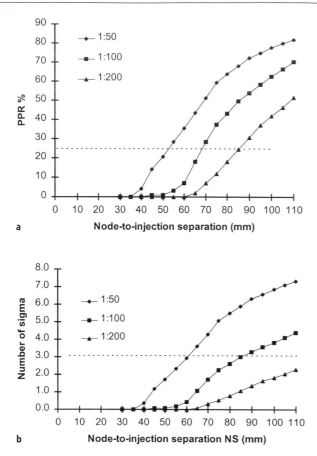

Fig. 3. **a** Example of the plot of percentage peak reduction (*PPR*) as the node-to-injection separation increases, for node-to-injection site activity ratios (NIR) of 1:50, 1:100 and 1:200. The 25% threshold is shown as a *dashed line*. The probe is N19; 5-mm-deep dual injection, 20-mm-deep node. **b** Plot of the number of standard deviations ($N\sigma$) in the difference between node peak *P* and minimum *M*, corresponding to the PPR plot in **a**. ISA, 2.5 MBq ^{99m}Tc. The 3σ threshold is shown as a *dashed line*

simulated profile and plotted as a function of NS for a given ISA and NIR (Fig. 3b). The separation at which a three sigma drop is achieved is referred to as MNS [3σ] and is read from this graph, allowing the statistical variation of the profile at any selected ISA and count rate to be investigated. Simulations were carried out at up to 110 mm NS, with the curve being linearly extrapolated to 115 mm, and the MNS [3σ] value read from the graph.

Results

Basic Physical Performance

There was no significant difference in cps/MBq between the probe sensitivity with the tip submerged beneath 20 mm water and that with the tip not submerged, with the source at 30 mm from the probe tip (mean difference 0.5%). Repeated sensitivity profiles with the N19 probe at 50 mm depth on different days, requiring re-clamping of the probe, showed mean variability of 2.9% in the cps/MBq sensitivity profile values. Sensitivity and spatial resolution (FWHM) values for the probes are given in Tables 1 and 2. Sensitivity falls by a factor of between 18 and 58 (mean 30) between 5 and 50 mm depth, whilst spatial resolution shows a factor of 3.5–5.3 (mean 4) increase in the FWHM as source depth increases from 5 to 50 mm. The probe depth error is estimated as ± 0.5 mm, leading to a maximum error of around ± 5% in the sensitivity measurement at 5 mm depth due to the rapid rate of change in sensitivity

Table 1. Sensitivity (cps/MBq) in relation to ^{99m}Tc source depth in water

Source depth (mm)	Probe				
	N19	N14	ECSI	ECDT	NAV
5	7310	6373	5752	3860	3770
10	4348	3989	2991	1495	1945
20	1740	1690	1170	363	787
30	924	895	592	188	396
50	350	350	226	66	143

Absolute error estimated as less than 10%; random error in each value estimated as less than 5.5%.

Table 2. Spatial resolution (mm) reported as the FWHM of the sensitivity profile, in relation to ^{99m}Tc source depth in water

Source depth (mm)	Probe				
	N19	N14	ECSI	ECDT	NAV
5	15.6	10.5	11.3	11.3	12.7
10	19.6	13.1	14.0	17.0	17.0
20	29.7	19.3	22.8	30.3	24.9
30	40.7	26.4	29.7	41.4	33.3
50	55.4	37.5	42.0	59.9	48.8

The error on each FWHM is estimated as less than 2.5 mm.

at 0 to 20 mm depth. The random error in sensitivity between different probes is therefore less than 5.5 % when the 2 % radioisotope calibrator variability is included, whilst the overall absolute sensitivity error is less than 10 % from the uncertainty in the radioisotope calibrator accuracy.

Validation

There was generally good agreement between the simulated and measured response to the two sources (Table 3), with a maximum error in the PPR of 5.3 % (Fig. 4). The error in PPR leads to an error in the MNS [25 %] values of approximately ± 3.5 mm when MNS [25 %] is read from the graph (see Fig. 3a).

Table 3. Comparison of simulated and experimental data

Probe	PPR (%)		
	Experimental data	Simulation	Error
N19	7.9	5.9	2.0
ECSI	49.6	54.8	– 5.3
ECDT	40.5	37.7	2.8

Two sources in water, one at 5 mm depth ("injection"), the other at 30 mm depth ("node"); NS, 80 mm; NIR, 1:60.

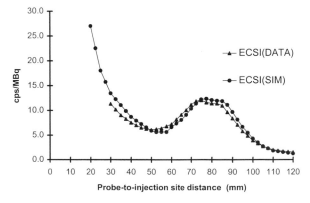

Fig. 4. Example of validation data for ECSI probe with two ^{99m}Tc sources. Experimental data [*ECSI(DATA)*] from 5-mm-deep ^{99m}Tc source ("injection") and 30-mm-deep ^{99m}Tc source ("node"); NIR, 1:60; NS, 80 mm. The simulated data are shown as *ECSI (SIM)*. These data show the maximum error magnitude in the PPR to be 5.3 %

Melanoma Simulation

Table 4 summarises the performance of the five probes in simulated localisation of a 30-mm-deep node with a 5-mm-deep dual injection site. The peak count rates at the minimum separation for statistical significance MNS [3σ] show a wide range between probes; for example, a factor of 6.3 from 40 cps (ECDT) to 253 cps (N14) at 1:50 NIR and 10 MBq in the injection site. With 1 MBq in the injection site at the time of localisation, no probe could identify the node if it was closer than 115 mm to the injection site, even at 1:50 NIR. With 2.5 MBq remaining in the injection site, ECDT could not localise the node at 1:50 NIR, and only N14 could localise it within 115 mm NS at 1:100. The N14 and ECSI probes were the only ones to reach 3σ within 115 mm separation with 10 MBq ISA and NIR 1:200.

The MNS [25 %] values were slightly lower for the ECSI probe than the N14 probe (6 mm, 7 mm and 10 mm better at NIR 1:50, 1:100 and 1:200, respectively, with an error in the comparison of ± 4.9 mm), and with less difference in MNS [3σ] (3 mm and 4 mm difference at 1:50 and 1:100), and almost the same performance at 1:200 NIR. The count rate from N14 was approximately 50 % higher than that from ECSI, but the final performance of these two probes was similar since the scatter sensitivity was lower for the ECSI probe. For example, with a 5-mm source depth the sensitivity at 30 mm off-axis as a percentage of the on-axis sensitivity was measured at 0.39 % for N14 and 0.23 % for ECSI.

Comparing the NAV and N19 probes, we see that NAV has slightly better MNS [3σ] (7 mm and 3 mm at NIR 1:50 and 1:100 respectively, at 10 MBq ISA), with count rates from N19 being 1.7 – 2 times that of the NAV probe. The ECDT probe has similar MNS [3σ] to N19 at NIR 1:50 and 10 MBq ISA, but with only one-fifth the count rate of N19.

Breast Simulation

The ability of the probes to localise nodes in the presence of deep injections (30 mm injection depth, 30-mm-deep node and 10 MBq ISA) is illustrated in Table 5. Performance is poorer than with 5-mm-deep injections, with the best MNS

Table 4. Probe performance in separating simulated 5-mm-deep injection site and 30-mm-deep node

| Probe | NIR | MNS [25%] (mm) | Injection site activity ISA (MBq) | | | |
| | | | 2.5 | | 10 | |
			MNS [3σ] (mm)	Peak cps	MNS [3σ] (mm)	Peak cps
N19	1:50	81	107	47	82	209
N14	1:50	54	69	56	54	253
ECSI	1:50	48	72	35	51	163
ECDT	1:50	62	>150	–	83	40
NAV	1:50	66	112	22	75	121
N19	1:100	102	>115	–	109	108
N14	1:100	69	113	26	76	127
ECSI	1:100	62	>115	–	72	82
ECDT	1:100	75	>115	–	>115	–
NAV	1:100	83	>115	–	106	55
N19	1:200	>115	>115	–	>115	–
N14	1:200	88	>115	–	110	61
ECSI	1:200	78	>115	–	112	41
ECDT	1:200	92	>115	–	>115	–
NAV	1:200	101	>115	–	>115	–

Minimum node-to-injection site separations, MNS, are shown based upon the requirement for a 25% fall from the node peak, MNS [25%], and the requirement that the fall reaches 3 standard deviations, MNS [3σ]. MNS [3σ] is given for 2.5 MBq and 10 MBq in the injection site. Peak cps is the count rate at the node peak. The errors in the minimum separation values MNS [25%] and MNS [3σ] are estimated.

Table 5. Probe performance from simulations of configuration related to breast tumour: single 30-mm-deep injection and 30-mm-deep node, with 10 MBq ISA

| Probe | MNS [25%] (mm) | | | MNS [3σ] (mm) | | |
	NIR 1:50	NIR 1:100	NIR 1:200	NIR 1:50	NIR 1:100	NIR 1:200
N19	102	>115	>115	103	>115	>115
N14	70	86	106	70	95	>115
ECSI	68	81	99	70	92	>115
ECDT	91	103	>115	>115	>115	>115
NAV	80	102	>115	92	>115	>115

[25%] value of 68 mm compared to 48 mm at 5 mm injection depth, and 10 MBq ISA is required to enable detection at 70 mm NS compared to 51 mm MNS [3σ] at 5 mm injection depth. The importance of counting statistics is highlighted by comparing the N19 and ECDT probes. The ECDT probe achieves a 25% PPR dip at 11 mm lower separations than N19 (91 vs 102 mm respectively), but with 10 MBq ISA the N19 probe reaches 3σ drop at 103 mm NS, whereas ECDT does not achieve a 3σ drop within 115 mm separation. This reflects the estimate that at the N19 node peak registers 209 cps, 5.2 times the expected 40 cps from the ECDT probe.

Probe Performance Ranking

The above considerations of shallow (5 mm) and deep (30 mm) injection with a 30-mm-deep node allow us to rank the probes in terms of the minimum node-to-injection site distance required to identify the node. The ranking is as follows in descending order of performance: ECSI and N14

Table 6. Minimum node-to-injection site separations (MNS) as node depth changes, all for 5-mm-deep dual injection. The probe is N19 with 2.5 MBq ISA

Node depth (mm)	MNS [25%] (mm)	MNS [3σ] (mm)
10	31	31
20	53	60
30	81	107

joint best, NAV, N19, ECDT. The best probes can identify nodes situated around 20–30 mm closer to the injection site than the poorest, and the ranking is the same for both the melanoma and breast injection simulations.

Node Depth Variation

As node depth increases the effects of reduced sensitivity (cps/MBq) and increasing FWHM of spatial resolution are shown for the N19 probe in Table 6, with rapidly increasing minimum separation required as node depth increases from 10 mm to 30 mm. The effects of reduced count rate at depth are highlighted at 30 mm node depth, where MNS [25%] is 81 mm, but statistical significance is not reached till the node is 107 mm, from the injection site at 2.5 MBq ISA. Conversely, these data also illustrate the rapid increase in localising ability as the probe approaches the node within the wound during surgery.

Changing the Lower Energy Threshold

Increasing the N19 lower energy threshold from 145 to 150 (arbitrary units) allows node localisation at around 3–4 mm lower NS values, whilst the 23% higher sensitivity at the lower threshold results in better localisation at 1:100 NIR with 2.5 MBq ISA.

Discussion

This work has shown that intra-operative gamma probe performance can be satisfactorily modelled from linear addition of basic sensitivity profiles.

Simulation allows objective comparison of probe performance in terms which directly relate to the task of identifying sentinel nodes in the presence of scatter from the injection site. Simulated data should be approached with caution to ensure that the necessary simplifications do not lead to unrealistic conclusions, and these simplifications are now discussed. Probes are simple radiation detectors, and allow linear addition of shifted data, as validated by this work. The model has to assume a certain standard geometry of probe, injection site and node for all different probe simulations. It is recognised that in practice angulation of the probe away from the injection site is widely used to reduce cross-talk, and though this angulation could easily be incorporated into the simulation, it offers no advantages in terms of comparative evaluation.

The model of the in vivo distribution of activity is relatively simple, but is adequate for the purpose of comparative probe evaluation. The node appears to be reasonably well represented by a small source, since mean node mass has been reported as 0.7±0.6 g [8], and most nodes are under 6 mm in maximum dimension [9]. The activity in the injection site is typically injected in 0.1 ml volume, and has been reported to reach a final volume in tissue of around 10 ml (8–12 ml) for antimony sulphur colloid [10]. If we assume that this volume is a hemisphere around the injection site then the radius of this hemisphere is 17 mm. This extended injection site activity will then require greater separation of the node before it is detectable, possibly of the order of 10 mm greater separation compared with an ideal point source. The idealised point source model therefore provides us with a "best-case" localisation, and poorer results must be expected in vivo. However, these differences in source size are not expected to affect relative ranking of probes since extended sources are merely linear additions of point sources. The model has mainly used a 30 mm node depth, being close to the mean node depth of 35 mm (range 10–80 mm) in the axilla [11], with 85% of internal mammary lymph nodes less than 30 mm deep [12], and with Yip and Ege [13] finding a mean internal mammary lymph node depth of 30 mm.

It is difficult to select a representative node-to-injection site activity ratio (NIR) since there is such a wide variation in radiocolloids and time delays between injection and operation, and even very wide variations given the same procedures. For example, with unfiltered ^{99m}Tc sulphur colloid in breast cancer, node uptake varies over three orders of magnitude, with a maximum of 0.28% of the injected dose at mean 3 h post injection [4]. Another study reported a median percentage of injected activity found in sentinel nodes of 0.36%, following intradermal injection of ^{99m}Tc-nano-colloid (Solco, Switzerland) and surgery at around 22 h delay [3]. Assuming little clearance from the injection site this gives a median NIR of around 1:280. The simulation has taken a range of NIRs from 1:50 to 1:200 to cover the limiting performance range of the probes for separating nodes within 110 mm of an injection site. Though this relatively high NIR range is valid for probe evaluation, future uses of this methodology to predict and optimise clinical use of the intra-operative probes will employ lower NIR values.

The simulation has not included a distributed background activity, since with operations at typically 3–24 h post injection the lymph channels and other tissues are relatively clear. Kapteijn et al. [3] have reported average skin and fat uptake per mass of tissue to be less than 1% of sentinel node uptake at around 22 h post ^{99m}Tc-nanocoll injection, whilst Albertini et al. [10] reported mean sentinel node-to-adjacent region count ratios of 39.2 at 2–4 h after injection of filtered ^{99m}Tc-sulphur colloid, and Mudun et al. [2] obtained ratios of 1:30 to 1:300 within a few hours of ^{99m}Tc-sulphur colloid injection.

To summarise these considerations of the model, the range of values we have used for model parameters will fall within the wide spectrum of conditions found in clinical practice, though tending to indicate better performance than will be met in vivo unless probe angulation is used. Further data will be of value in improving the simulation as a description of clinical performance, but are unlikely to change the relative ranking of the probe systems.

To compare probe performance, we set a percentage peak reduction (PPR) of 25% from the node peak and three standard deviations of difference as selection criteria. The 25% threshold was set based upon laboratory experience with test sources, with the judgement that the systems gave sufficient feedback to the user, both audibly and through the count rate display, to identify a 25% change. Little change would be expected in the overall ranking of the five probes tested here if a different PPR threshold were to be set since the rates of change of PPR per millimetre node-to-injection site separation are very similar between different probes. That is, if the threshold PPR value changes then the absolute values of the minimum separations will change, though differences between probes will tend to be preserved.

The motivation for this work was the difficulty experienced in evaluating and ranking probes from the basic physical performance data of sensitivity and spatial resolution. Given the basic data, can we say which probe is best, and does this agree with the ranking achieved through the simulation analysis? Consider first the basic physical data. The N14 probe has the best spatial resolution and the second best sensitivity, whilst the ECSI probe has slightly poorer spatial resolution and poorer sensitivity. The ECDT and NAV probes have similar sensitivities at 5 mm depth, with NAV maintaining sensitivity at greater depths due to the lower energy threshold used (95 versus 110 keV). Spatial resolution is generally poorer for ECDT than for NAV. The N19 probe is harder to rank on basic physical performance data since it has the highest spatial sensitivity but is at the low end of spatial resolution, similar to ECDT. In summary, the basic physical performance data might lead us to conclude that the N14 probe is best, followed by the ECSI probe. Similarly, ECDT should be the poorest, whilst the relative ranking of NAV and N19 is not clear. This is to be compared with the results of the simulation analysis, which show that there is no significant difference between the technical performance of N14 and ECSI probes in the task of sentinel node localisation, though the basic performance comparison had led us to expect N14 to be superior to ECSI. NAV then performs next best, followed by N19 and ECDT. We see that the simulation evaluation of these five probes leads to a change in ranking for the top two probes, and allows NAV and N19 to be ranked. In addition to changed and clearer ranking, the simulation provides a clear measure of how the performance will practically differ, showing that the best-performing probes will be able to identify nodes up to 30 mm closer to the injection site than will be achieved with the poorest probes.

Limitations arise from the basic performance data since they are reported as summary parameters: the FWHM of the spatial sensitivity profile and the sensitivity on-axis. In practice we have seen that the limiting performance is more closely related to the tails of the sensitivity profile at the 1% or lower level, and so a wide range of the sensitivity profile determines performance. We note that the main source of overlap between the injection source and the node source is through scatter. This is seen since minimum separations between node and injection site are at least 50 mm, for a 5-mm-deep injection source, with the minimum dip in counts around 30 mm from the injection site. With this geometry only scattered radiation is detected from the injection site, with very little direct penetration through the probe collimation. Evaluation of probe performance therefore requires measurement of the sensitivity at distances well beyond the FWHM values, and measurements at up to at least 120 mm off-axis are required.

Each probe requires optimisation of lower energy thresholds or energy windows, altering sensitivity and scatter rejection. The simulation method shows how optimisation may be objectively performed, with the example of increasing the N19 lower threshold from 145 to 150 (arbitrary units) showing some advantages of higher sensitivity at the lower threshold in finding low uptake nodes, despite higher scatter acceptance. Other probe features such as different collimation could be optimised using the same approach.

This numerical simulation has not been able to include other factors which may influence overall performance as perceived by the operator. For example, though the N14 probe requires slightly greater node separation than ECSI in all cases, N14 also delivers approximately 50% higher count rate. It is not known whether this higher count rate, and lower statistical variation, will be perceived by the operator as more reliable than the lower ECSI count rate, even though the greater scatter rejection of the ECSI probe enables it to match the N14 performance at lower count rates. In very low uptake nodes, such as those found with large colloid particle size [4], and remote from the injection site such that cross-talk is reduced, sensitivity may be the dominant performance factor, though further studies are required to investigate this.

In overall system evaluation other factors such as visual display clarity, audible feedback, size and weight of probes and dynamic range must also be taken into account and clinical testing of probes is always recommended.

Conclusions

A simulation technique has been presented and validated which enables the practical performance of intra-operative gamma probes to be evaluated specifically for the task of sentinel node localisation. This is illustrated with comparison of five probe systems, showing clear differences in expected practical performance. The technique could be useful for system optimisation and user education, and allows ranking of probe systems in an objective manner based upon data directly related to the probe performance in sentinel node localisation.

■ **Acknowledgements.** I thank Mr. Barry Powell for the use of an intra-operative probe, Mr. Stephen Anderson of Bright Technologies for loan of a probe, and Mr. Doug Cookson of Neoprobe for the loan of probes. To Mr. Ron Clark and Mr. Chris Keyte thanks for workshop support, and to Dr. Dariush Nassiri thanks for loan of the positioning frame.

References

1. Alazraki NP, Eshima D, Eshima LA et al. Lymphoscintigraphy, the sentinel node concept and the intraoperative gamma probe in melanoma, breast cancer and other potential cancers. *Semin Nucl Med* 1997; 27:55–67
2. Mudun A, Murray DR, Herda SC, Eshima D, Shattuck LA, Vansant JP, Taylor AT, Alazraki NP. Early stage melanoma: lymphoscintigraphy, reproducibility of sentinel node detection, and effectiveness of the intraoperative gamma probe. *Radiology* 1996; 199:171–175
3. Kapteijn BAE, Nieweg OE, Muller SH, Liem IH, Hoefnagel CA, Rutgers EJTh, Kroon BBR. Validation of gamma probe detection of the sentinel node in melanoma. *J Nucl Med* 1997; 38:362–366
4. Gulec SA, Moffatt FL, Carroll RG, Serafini AN, Sfakianakis GN, Allen L, Boggs J, Escobedo D, Pruett CS, Gupta A, Livingstone AS, Krag DN. Sentinel lymph node localisation in early breast cancer. *J Nucl Med* 1998; 39:1388–1393
5. Veronesi U, Paganelli G, Galimberti V, Viale G, Zurrida S, Bedoni M, Costa A, de Cicco C, Geraghty JG, Luini A, Sacchini V, Veronesi P. Sentinel node biopsy to avoid axillary dissection in breast cancer with clinically negative lymph-nodes. *Lancet* 1997; 349:1864–1867
6. Tiorina T, Arends B, Huysmans D, Rutten H, Lemaire B, Muller S. Evaluation of surgical gamma pobes for radioguided sentinel node localisation. *Eur J Nucl Med* 1998; 25:1224–1231

7. Waddington WA, Davidson BR, Todd-Pokropek A, Boulos PB, Short MD. Evaluation of a technique for the intra-operative detection of a radiolabelled monoclonal antibody against colorectal cancer. *Eur J Nucl Med* 1991; 18: 964–972

8. Bergqvist L, Strand SE, Persson B, Hafstrom L, Jonsson PE. Dosimetry in lymphoscintigraphy of Tc-99m antimony sulfur colloid. *J Nucl Med* 1982; 23:698–705

9. Collier DB, Palmer DW, Wilson JF, Greenberg M, Komaki R, Cox JD, Lawson TL, Lawlor PM. Internal mammary lymphoscintigraphy in patients with breast cancer. *Radiology* 1983; 147:845–848

10. Albertini JJ, Lyman GH, Cox C, Yeatman T, Balducci L, Ku N, Shivers S, Berman C, Wells K, Rapaport D, Shons A, Horton J, Greenberg H, Nicosia S, Clark R, Cantor A, Reintgen DS. Lymphatic mapping and sentinel node biopsy in the patient with breast cancer. *JAMA* 1996; 276:1818–1822

11. Uren RF, Howman-Giles RB, Thompson JF, Malouf D, Ramsey-Stewart G, Niesche FW, Renwick SB. Mammary lymphoscintigraphy in breast cancer. *J Nucl Med* 1995; 36:1775–1780

12. Kaplan WD, Andersen JW, Siddon RL, Connolly BT, McCormick CA, Laffin SM, Rosenbaum EM, Jennings CA, Recht A, Harris JR. The three dimensional localization of internal mammary lymph nodes by radionuclide lymphoscintigraphy. *J Nucl Med* 1988; 29:473–478

13. Yip TC, Ege GN. Determination of the depth distribution of the internal mammary lymph nodes on lateral lymphoscintigraphy. *Clin Radiol* 1985; 36:149–152

CHAPTER 5

Injection Techniques

Breast Carcinoma

There is as yet no single accepted method for sentinel node localisation, and there are significant variations in the injection technique used for the administration of radionuclide colloids. The techniques range from single subdermal injection [1] to multiple peritumoral [2–6] and even intratumoral injection [7]. Other variables (described elsewhere in the book) include the type of colloidal particles used, with special emphasis on particle size [8] and the volume [9, 10] of the injectate. In brief, with a small particle size the risk of sampling non-sentinel nodes is increased due to spill-over of the colloid to other nodes, leading to sampling of an increased number of lymph nodes [3, 11]; on the other hand, with a larger particle size the transport may be inadequate, resulting in a higher sentinel node detection failure rate. Despite variation in the techniques used for sentinel node localisation, the overall results are encouraging. In a recent combined analysis by McMasters and co-workers [12], in 1385 patients with breast carcinoma the overall sensitivity was 94 % and the specificity 100 % when the sentinel node histology was compared with the axillary node dissection specimen. The overall accuracy reported in this combined analysis was 98 %, with a positive predictive value of 100 % and a negative predictive value of 97 % (Table 1).

There is nevertheless significant variation in the rate of detection of internal mammary lymph nodes and this seems to be dependent on the mode of administration of the colloid. The subdermal injection technique is associated with the lowest detection rate of internal mammary nodes, and higher detection rates are reported with an intratumoral and a peritumoral approach.

It is the aim of this chapter to describe the practical aspects of various injection techniques.

Palpable Breast Carcinoma

Patient Selection

The patient selection criteria for the sentinel node biopsy trial conducted at our Institution for breast cancer are as follows:

Eligibility Criterion:

1. Proven palpable or non-palpable invasive carcinoma of the breast on "triple assessment", i.e. clinical examination, imaging (mammogram and ultrasound) and tissue diagnosis (cytology, Tru-cut biopsy), where surgical treatment would involve removal of the primary tumour and axillary dissection

Table 1. Studies of sentinel node biopsy with concommitant axillary dissection in patients with breast cancer (from McMasters et al. [12])

Study	No. of patients	Pts with SLN identified no. (%)	Technique	Sensitivity (%)	Specificity (%)	Positive predictive value (%)	Negative predictive value (%)	Overall accuracy (%)	SLN only positive node (%)	False-negative rate (%)
All	1385	1198 (86)	All	94	100	100	97	98	48	6.2

SLN, Sentinel lymph node.

Exclusion Criteria:

1. Pregnancy/lactation
2. Previous breast or axillary surgery at the same site
3. Multifocal/multicentric carcinomas of the breast
4. Clinical involvement of the axillary lymph node(s)

At our Institution a subdermal injection is used in most patients, although in those with large breasts and a deeply situated carcinoma the injection is given into the breast parenchyma in a peritumoral fashion. Previous breast surgery should not be regarded as an absolute contraindication to sentinel node biopsy. It seems that the success rate of sentinel node localisation is lower in patients with previous breast surgery [4] but that the false-negative rate is not affected [5].

Multifocal tumours are likely to involve more than one lymphatic trunk from the mammary gland to the axillary nodes, giving rise to a false-negative result [1,13]. Two out of four false-negative cases in a study performed by Veronesi et al. [1] had multifocal tumours, and other groups have also reported false-negative results because of multifocality of the primary breast cancer [14]. It is very important to exclude those patients with clinical suspicion of axillary lymph node involvement. This is one of the potential pitfalls in sentinel node localisation [5] and can lead to a false-negative result. This is likely to be due to a change in the lymphatic flow if the sentinel node is replaced with metastatic carcinoma and is mechanically blocked and non-functional; as a result of the flow changes, the colloid bypasses the sentinel node and moves on to a non-sentinel lymph node. This point is clearly demonstrated in case no. 22 in Chap. 11.

Preparation for Injection

It is good practice to explain the procedure in detail to the patient and to obtain informed consent. In particular it is important to mention that this technique in breast cancer management is at present under investigation and research. The injection can be administered the day prior to surgery or on the day of the operation in accordance with the agreed protocol. It is important to check the total dose and the volume of technetium-99m colloid (Fig. 1a). It is good radiation safety practice to be ready to inject (Fig. 1b) before removing the

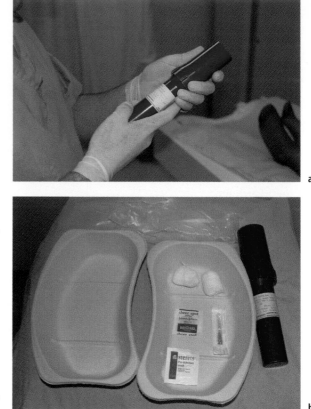

Fig. 1. a The volume and dose of ^{99m}Tc-colloid are checked before administration. **b** Materials are prepared before handling the radionuclide

syringe from its lead case, and a syringe shield may also be used for this purpose. The injection time and the dose and mode of injection need to be recorded carefully.

Subdermal Injection

The subdermal injection technique was described by Veronesi and co-workers [1], who successfully detected the sentinel nodes in 98% of 163 patients using a combination of lymphoscintigraphy and a gamma probe after subdermal injection of ^{99m}Tc-colloidal albumin. This technique is based on the fact that the breast is developmentally derived from the ectoderm [15]. The dermal and parenchymal lymphatics of the breast meet at the subareolar lymphatic plexus [16] and from here one to two main lymphatic trunks drain towards the axilla (Fig. 2). Sappey's illustration of one or two large collecting lymph trunks originating from the subareolar lymphatic plexus has been

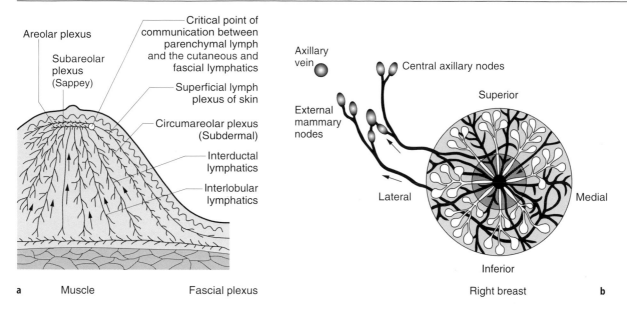

Fascial plexus   Right breast   **b**

Fig. 2. a According to Sappey, all lymph from breast drains into the subareolar plexus. **b** Demonstration of the critical point of communication between parenchymal and cutaneous lymphatics. (Modified from Grant RN et al. [16])

confirmed by other investigators using direct lymphangiographic techniques [17, 18].

Borgstein and co-workers [15] confirmed the hypothesis that the lymphatics of the overlying skin drain to the same axillary sentinel node as the underlying glandular breast tissue. They injected radioactive colloid into the breast parenchyma in a peritumoral fashion in 33 consecutive females with invasive breast cancer and in the operating room the blue dye was injected intradermally. There was a 100% concordance in delineation of the sentinel node with intradermal blue dye and with intra-mammary ^{99m}Tc-labelled albumin. The location of the primary tumour and the tumour size seemed not to alter the success rate of the procedure. The advantages of the subdermal technique are that it is more predictable and rapid, and has a high success rate in localising the sentinel node owing to the very rich subdermal lymphatic plexus.

■ **The Subdermal Injection Procedure.** The day preceding surgery, a single dose of 10–15 MBq of ^{99m}Tc-labelled Albures or Nanocoll is injected subdermally (Fig. 3) at the tumour site, using a 25-G needle and a volume of 0.2 ml. The Albures prepa-

ration we have used has a particle size of less than 400 nm, whilst at present, Nanocoll has a particle size of less than 80 nm, with 90% of particles being between 30 and 40 nm.

The patient is positioned in a supine position with the arm to the side. The tumour is palpated and the overlying skin carefully marked. The

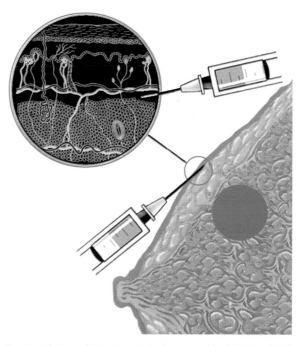

Fig. 3. Subdermal injection technique. 0.2 ml of ^{99m}Tc-colloid with 0.2 ml of air behind it is injected in the subdermal lymphatic plexus

tracer dose of 10–15 MBq of colloid in a volume of 0.2 ml is prepared such that 0.2 ml of air is drawn into the syringe behind the radioactive colloid. The main purpose of this is to ensure that no radiocolloid is left in the needle after the injection, as the volume of the injectate is small. This also safeguards against spillage of the radiocolloid, which may cause a contamination artefact after withdrawal of the needle, mimicking the sentinel node (see case no. 8 in Chap. 11). The other advantage of an air bubble in the syringe is that it helps to disperse the colloid in the subdermal space. Figure 4 clearly demonstrates the first point. In this case air was not drawn into the syringe and on withdrawing the plunger after the injection had been given, approximately half of the injection dose was left in the syringe.

The syringe is held at an angle of 10–20° to the horizontal plane and the skin overlying the tumour is punctured using a 25-G needle (Fig. 5). The injection is delivered to the subdermal lymphatic plexus and this is confirmed by a raised bleb at the injection site. After the injection has been given, cotton wool is applied over the injection site, and to prevent back-flow of the injected colloid and skin contamination the injection site is sealed

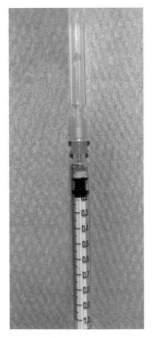

Fig. 4. Case demonstrating the importance of an air bubble in the syringe for subdermal injection. Half of the injection dose was retained in the needle

using a small adhesive plaster. The patient is asked to massage over the injection site for a minute with fresh cotton wool.

It is the responsibility of the physician administering the radiopharmaceutical to ensure the proper disposal of the waste.

Peritumoral Injection

Peritumoral injection is a commonly practiced method of injection of the radiopharmaceutical. The radiocolloid is injected around the tumour into the breast parenchyma (Fig. 6).

This technique differs from the subdermal technique in that the removal of the tracer and the dye is slower due to the scantier lymphatic supply of the breast parenchyma [5, 19]. In this setting, dynamic imaging is less useful since one is less likely to see the lymphatic tract. Imaging is commonly performed 1–2 h after the injection has been administered.

■ **The Peritumoral Injection Technique.** The skin is penetrated with the syringe held vertically and a larger injection volume is given with this technique (Fig. 7). The injection is usually given at four sites, superior, inferior, medial and lateral to the tumour. Krag et al. [20] have emphasized the importance of the volume of the radiocolloid injectate in the success of this technique. They proposed that a volume of 4–8 ml in four 1- to 2-ml aliquots is optimal. Some investigators inject around a 180° arc facing the axillary side of the primary tumour.

Intratumoral Injection

The intratumoral injection technique is not widely used and it appears that at present only one centre is practising this technique [7]. Concerns have been expressed with regard to direct injection into a high-pressure tumour environment and there are also theoretical worries about tumour dissemination and needle tract seeding. For this technique to be acceptable for routine clinical practice, there must be a clear advantage over other available techniques and such an advantage is not evident at present.

Non-palpable Breast Carcinoma

With widespread use of screening mammography and increased patient awareness, an increasing

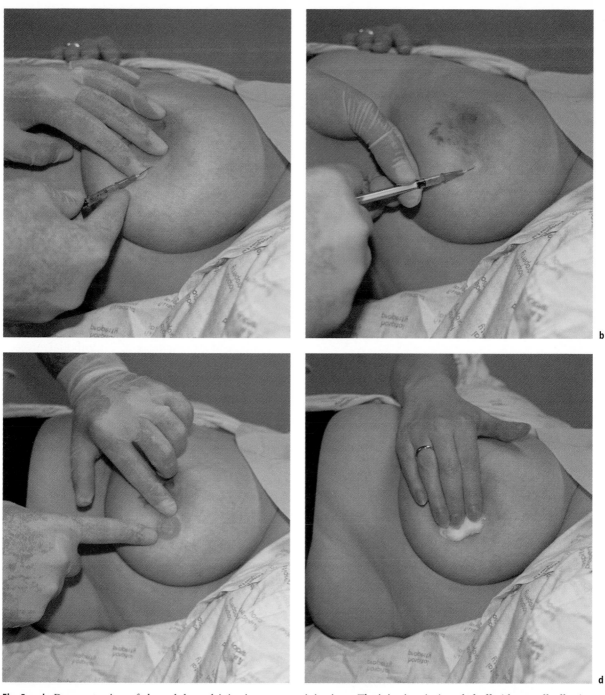

Fig. 5 a–d. Demonstration of the subdermal injection steps. **a** The needle is held parallel to the breast and the skin overlying the tumour is punctured. **b** A bleb is raised during injection. **c** The injection site is sealed off with a small adhesive plaster. **d** The patient is asked to gently massage over the injection area

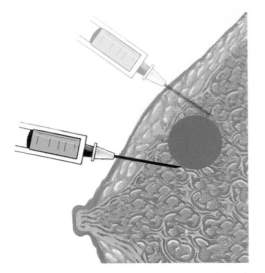

Fig. 6. Peritumoral injection technique. The radionuclide is delivered into the breast parenchyma. A larger volume of injectate is used and it is usually delivered in multiple sites around the tumour

number of non-palpable screen-detected breast carcinomas are seen. Since they represent early breast carcinoma, these lesions are the most suitable for sentinel node biopsy. However, a definitive diagnosis of invasive breast carcinoma is mandatory before considering these patients for sentinel node biopsy.

In the case of superficial non-palpable lesions that are detected by ultrasound scan, the overlying skin can be marked by the radiologist, and the injection can be given subdermally at the

Fig. 7 a, b. Peritumoral injection. The syringe is held perpendicular to skin and the radiopharmaceutical is delivered around the primary tumour

marked site with the technique described above. For deeper lesions that require needle localisation prior to excision, the radiopharmaceutical can be given in the radiology department under image guidance (Fig. 8) The position of the needle is verified before the injection is administered.

Kinetics of ^{99m}Tc-Labelled Colloid

Lymphatic capillaries are lined by endothelial cells which overlap each other to a varying degree. Unlike the vascular endothelium, the lymphatic endothelial cells do not rest upon a continuous basal membrane. Instead they are suspended within surrounding interstitial tissue by longitudinal bundles of collagen fibres called "anchoring filaments". These anchoring filaments occur at regular intervals over the lymphatic vessel wall, and they are seen on surfaces of endothelial projections and overlapping terminal margins of adjacent endothelial cells, which are called patent junctions [21]. As a result of increased interstitial fluid volume in the connective tissue, traction is exerted on the fibres, resulting in passive separation of adjacent endothelial cells [22]. Entrance of particles and tumour cells into the lymphatics is gained through the patent junctions. It appears that the radiolabelling efficacy of sentinel node localisation in breast cancer using an intramammary injection technique is closely related to the injection volume. Krag's multicentre trial group have reported that injection of a larger volume of the radiopharmaceutical is required to facilitate lymphatic uptake through maximal distention of

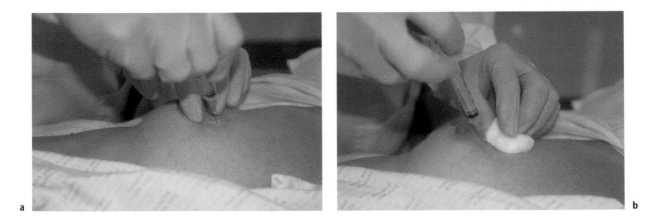

a   b

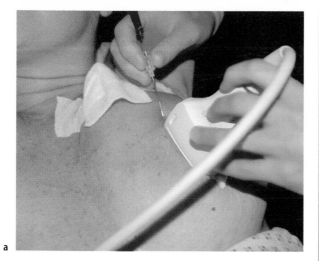

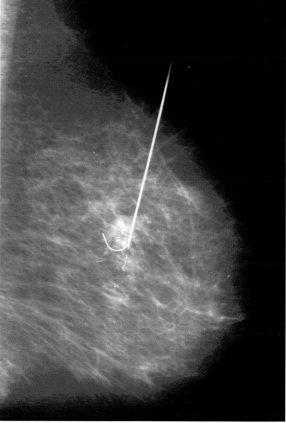

Fig. 8. In non-palpable breast carcinoma the radionuclide can be injected during ultrasound-guided localisation (**a**) or mammography-guided localisation (**b**)

anchoring filaments. Sentinel node identification rates were 96 % and 100 % with 4-cc and 8-cc injection volumes respectively [20].

Many lymphatic collateral vessels are present, but they only become accessible if there is change in flow and valve incompetence due to distal obstruction. In this way the lymphatic flow and spread of tumour may become retrograde and unpredictable. Gilchrist demonstrated this through an experiment by injecting coloured particles under increasing pressure: there was a change in the direction and rerouting of lymphatic flow through proximal collateral channels to reach retrograde nodes [23].

Malignant Melanoma

The sentinel node technique is widely accepted as an accurate staging procedure in malignant melanoma, and it has almost replaced elective lymph node dissection. Sentinel node biopsy has been suggested as a standard of care in management of melanoma patients [24].

Injection Technique

The injection technique is similar to the subdermal injection technique described for breast cancer. On the day before or on the same day as surgery, 15 MBq of colloid is injected subdermally in a volume of 0.2 ml. If the primary lesion is still present, the injection is administered around it. In patients who have undergone previous excision biopsy, the injection is divided into four equal portions of 0.2 ml and administered on each side of biopsy scar, about 5 mm away from the wound edge, using a 25-G needle (Fig. 9). The syringe is held parallel to the skin surface and the needle enters at an angle of 10 – 20° to the horizontal plane (Fig. 9). Again, it is useful to draw some air into the syringe for the reasons already explained.

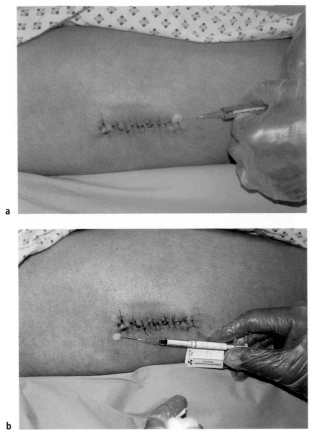

Fig. 9 a, b. Injection technique in malignant melanoma. This patient had undergone previous excision biopsy

As by definition the sentinel node has the highest chance of tumour involvement, lymphatic mapping and sentinel node biopsy in this setting potentially enhances the detection of micrometastases. This is achieved by careful examination of the sentinel node, including immunohistochemistry and the reverse-transcriptase polymerase chain reaction (RT-PCR).

The clinical significance of micrometastases in colorectal cancer has been reported by Liefers et al. [27]. These authors analysed 192 lymph nodes from 26 consecutive patients with stage II colorectal cancer using carcinoembryonic antigen-specific nested RT-PCR. Micrometastases were detected in 14 of 26 patients (54%). The adjusted 5-year survival rate for cancer-related death was 50% in this group as compared with 91% in the 12 patients without micrometastases. The authors conclude that diagnosis of micrometastases in stage II colorectal cancer is a prognostic tool. Moreover, in a feasibility study by Saha et al. on 30 consecutive patients with 25 colon and five rectal carcinomas [28], sentinel node mapping successfully predicted the lymph node status of the lymphatic basin in 28 (93.3%). In 4/30 (13.3%) the sentinel node was the only site of metastasis; this may have up-staged these patients, who could then potentially benefit from implementation of adjuvant therapy. Additional lymph node metastases beyond the usual site may be identified, and thus may alter the surgical resection margin. In the aforementioned study by Saha et al. there were no significant complications as a result of blue dye injection except in one patient who developed transient hypotension without any deleterious effect.

In patients who have previously undergone wide excision, the injection can be administered into the subdermal lymphatic plexus at four sites around the wide excision, in the 3, 6, 9 and 12 o'clock positions. However, it is noted that very wide excision of primary melanoma is regarded as an exclusion criterion by some groups since the altered lymphatic drainage following wide excision [25] increases the failure rate of sentinel node detection [26].

Colorectal Cancer

The sentinel node concept can also be extended to colorectal carcinoma as well. If there is no metastatic involvement of the lymph nodes, colorectal cancer patients are not treated with adjuvant chemotherapy. Nevertheless, more than 30% of such patients subsequently go on to develop recurrence.

Injection Technique

Patients with proven colorectal cancer can be included. At operation 2 ml of patent blue dye is injected subserosally around the tumour (Fig. 10). Care is taken not to spill the blue dye during the injection as this can cause blue discoloration of the surrounding tissue and can make sentinel node detection difficult. Usually the blue node(s) can be identified within 5 min of injection, during which time the mobilisation of the bowel can continue. The blue sentinel node can then be

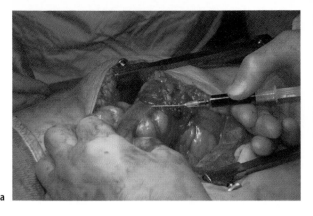

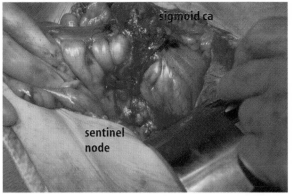

Fig. 10 a, b. Injection technique in colon cancer using patent blue dye. The dye is injected in the subserosal plane

marked with a suture, and the dissection continued further.

It is our experience that with rectal carcinoma it is more feasible to inject the patent blue dye submucosally around the tumour using a proctoscope (Fig. 11a). The drawback of this technique is that by the time the rectum is fully mobilised, the blue dye has progressed through most of the mesorectal nodes (Fig. 11b). The sentinel node can be identified by careful ex vivo dissection of the mesorectum to identify the first blue node that is closest to the primary tumour. Further work is required to optimise this technique.

Fig. 11. In rectal carcinoma the blue dye can be injected submucosally around the tumour by using a proctoscope whilst the patient is under general anaesthesia (**a**). The resected specimen demonstrates that the blue dye travels along the lymphatic chain. The closest blue node to the tumour can be marked as the sentinel node (**b**)

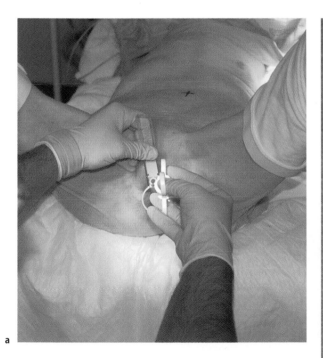

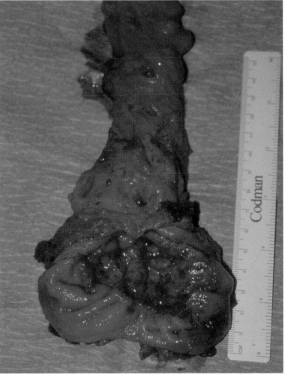

Penile Cancer

It is worth mentioning that the sentinel node was first described by Cabanas [29] in the management of penile cancer patients, more than 20 years ago. This work was based on the concept of sequential dissemination of the tumour cells and the hypothesis that identification of tumour cells in the sentinel node would indicate the need for lymph node dissection. Cabanas performed lymphangiography via dorsal lymphatics of the penis and labelled the node in proximity to the superficial epigastric vein as a sentinel node.

Injection Technique

Lymphoscintigraphy is preceded by subdermal injection of 15 MBq of ^{99m}Tc-nanocolloid in a volume of 0.2 ml around the tumour. As injection in this site can be very painful, prior application of topical anaesthetic may be helpful. Use of the needle-free syringe may be ideal for this condition (see Chap. 14). If the primary tumour has been excised by circumcision, the injection can be administered on the dorsum of the penis, proximal to the corona (Fig. 12). This is followed by dynamic imaging as described in Chap. 6.

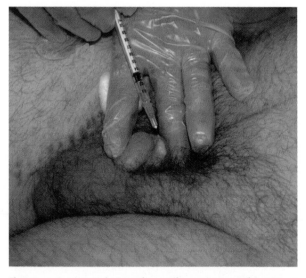

Fig. 12. Injection technique for penile carcinoma. This patient had previously been circumcised as part of his treatment

Key Points for Clinical Practice

- Despite variation in the technique for administration of colloids, excellent results of sentinel node localisation biopsy have been reported.
- The subdermal injection technique for breast cancer is a fast and reliable technique with a good success rate for sentinel node localisation.
- Upon peritumoral injection in breast carcinoma, the flow of tracer is slower due to reduced lymphatics in the breast parenchyma; accordingly a larger volume of the injectate at multiple sites is required for this technique to be successful.
- The rate of internal mammary identification varies with the injection technique; it seems to be lowest with a subdermal technique.
- Patients with clinical involvement of the axilla or multifocal breast cancer should be excluded from sentinel node biopsy since these conditions are associated with a higher false-negative rate.
- Previous surgery to the breast is accompanied by a reduced rate of detection of the sentinel node but the false-negative rate is not increased.
- Spillage of radiopharmaceutical must be avoided during injection as it leads to contamination artefact and difficulty in interpretation of the image.
- Good radiation safety procedures should always be observed during administration of radio-colloid.
- Detection of the sentinel node is highly accurate in melanoma and breast cancer.
- The technique can be better optimised through a large well-designed multicentre trial.
- Sentinel node localisation requires a multidisciplinary approach and its success depends on good teamwork.

References

1. Veronesi U, Paganelli G, Galimberti V, Viale G, Zurrida ST, Bodeni N, Costa A, Chicco C, Geraghty JG, Luine A, Sacchini V, Veronesi P. *Lancet* 1997; 349:1864–1867
2. Alex JC, Krag DN. The gamma-probe-guided resection of radiolabeled primary lymph nodes. *Surg Oncol Clin North Am* 1996; 5:33–41
3. Uren RF, Howman-Giles RB, Thompson JF, Malouf D, Ramsey-Stewart G, Niesche FW, Renwick SB. Mammary lymphoscintigraphy in breast cancer. *J Nucl Med* 1995; 36:1775–1780

4. Albertini JJ, Lyman GH, Cox C, Yeatman T, Balducci L, Ku N, Shivers S, Berman C, Wells K, Rapaport D, Shons A, Horton J, Greenberg H, Nicosia S, Clark R, Cantor A, Reintgen DS. Lymphatic mapping and sentinel node biopsy in the patient with breast cancer. *JAMA* 1996; 276:1818–1822

5. Borgstein PJ, Pijpers R, Comans EF, van Diest PJ, Boom RP, Meijer S. Sentinel lymph node biopsy in breast cancer: guidelines and pitfalls of lymphoscintigraphy and gamma probe detection. *J Am Coll Surg* 1998; 186:275–283

6. Crossin JA, Johnson AC, Stewart PB, Turner WW Jr. Gamma-probe-guided resection of the sentinel lymph node in breast cancer. *Am Surg* 1998; 64:666–668

7. Kapteijn BAE, Nieweg OE, Peterse JL, Rutgers EJTh, Hart AAM, van Dongen JA, Kroon BBR. *Identification and biopsy of the sentinel node in breast cancer*. Academisch Proefschrift, Universität of Amsterdam

8. Bergqvist L, Strand S-E, Persson BRR. Particle sizing and biokinetics of interstitial lymphoscintigraphic agents. *Semin Nucl Med* 1983; 13:9–19

9. Pijpers R, Meijer S, Hoekstra OS et al. Impact of lymphoscintigraphy on sentinel node identification with technetium-99m colloidal albumin in breast cancer. *J Nucl Med* 1997; 38:366–368

10. Pijpers R, Collet GJ, Meijer S, Hoekstra OS. The impact of dynamic lymphoscintigraphy and gamma probe guidance on sentinel node biopsy in melanoma. *Eur J Nucl Med* 1995; 22:1238–1241

11. McCarthy WH, Thompson JF, Uren RF. Invited commentary. *Arch Surg* 1995; 130:659

12. McMasters KM, Giuliano AE, Ross MI et al. Sentinel-lymph-node biopsy for breast cancer – not yet the standard of care. *N Engl J Med* 1998; 339:990–995

13. Veronesi U, Zurrida S, Galimberti V. Consequences of sentinel node in clinical decision making in breast cancer and prospects for future studies. *Eur J Surg Oncol* 1998; 24:93–95

14. O'Hea BJ, Hill AD, El-Shirbiny AM, Yeh SD, Rosen PP, Coit DG, Borgen PI, Cody HS. Sentinel lymph node biopsy in breast cancer: initial experience at Memorial Sloan-Kettering Cancer Center. *J Am Coll Surg* 1998; 186:423–427

15. Borgstein PJ, Meijer S, Pijpers R. Intradermal blue dye to identify sentinel lymph-node in breast cancer. *Lancet* 1997; 349:1668–1669

16. Grant RN, Tabah EJ, Adair FE. The surgical significance of the subareolar plexus in cancer of the breast. *Surgery* 1959; 33:71–78

17. Halsell JT, Smith JR, Bentlage CR, Park OK, Humphreys JW. Lymphatic drainage of the breast demonstrated by vital dye staining and radiography. *Ann Surg* 1965; 162:221–226

18. Kett K, Varga G, Lukacs L. Direct lymphography of the breast. *Lymphology* 1970; 1:3–12

19. Gulec SA, Moffat FL, Carroll RG, Serafini AN, Sfakianakis GN, Allen L, Boggs J, Escobedo D, Pruett CS, Gupta A, Livingstone AS, Krag DN. Sentinel lymph node localization in early breast cancer. *J Nucl Med* 1998; 39:1388–1393

20. Krag DN, Ashikaga T, Harlow SP, Weaver DI. Development of sentinel node targeting technique in breast cancer patients. *Breast* 1998; 4:67–74

21. Gulec SA, Moffat FL, Carroll RG, Krag DN. Gamma probe guided sentinel node biopsy in breast cancer. *Q J Nucl Med* 1997; 41:251–261

22. Leak LV. Electron microscopic observations on lymphatic capillaries and the structural components of the connective tissue-lymph interface. *Microvasc Res* 1970; 2:361–391

23. Gilchrist RK. Fundamental factors governing lymphatic spread of carcinoma. *Ann Surg* 1940; 111:630–639

24. Reintgen DS. Changing standards of surgical care for melanoma patients. *Ann Surg Oncol* 1996; 14:7–17

25. Rees WV, Robinson DS, Holmes EC, Morton DL. Altered lymphatic drainage following lymphadenectomy. *Cancer* 1980; 45:3045–3049

26. Morton DL, Wen DR, Wong JH, Economou JS, Cagle LA, Storm FK, Foshag LJ, Cochran AJ. Technical details of intraoperative lymphatic mapping for early stage melanoma. *Arch Surg* 1992; 127:392–399

27. Liefers GJ, Cleton-Jansen AM, van de Velde CJ, Hermans J, van Krieken, Cornelisse CJ, Tollenar RA. Micrometastases and survival in grade II colorectal cancer. *N Engl J Med* 1998; 339:223–228

28. Saha S, Espinosa M, Gauthier J, Morrison A, Rohatgi C, Dorman S. Ganatra BK, Desai D, Arora M. *Diagnostic and therapeutic implications of sentinel node mapping in colorectal cancer*. 51st Society of Surgical Oncology, 1st World Federation of Surgical Oncology Societies Cancer Symposium, San Diego, Calif, March 26–29, 1998: 31

29. Cabanas R. An approach for the treatment of penile carcinoma. *Cancer* 1977; 39:456–466

CHAPTER 6

Imaging Techniques

Introduction

Worldwide a number of groups are currently evaluating, refining and establishing the sentinel node biopsy technique as clinical practice. The pioneering work of Morton introduced intra-operative lymphatic mapping by injection of a vital blue dye into tissue surrounding the tumour, thereby enabling detection of the sentinel node visually by dissection along the blue-stained afferent lymphatic vessel to the first draining node [1]. An alternative approach was developed by Krag and co-workers [2–4], who detected the sentinel node after the injection of a radiolabelled colloid by means of a hand-held surgical gamma detecting probe. The pattern of lymphatic drainage of a radiocolloidal tracer in melanoma has been imaged pre-operatively both as an initial step in the radionuclide-guided detection of the sentinel node [5, 6] and as a complement to the technique of intra-operative lymphatic mapping [1, 7].

Sentinel node imaging is regarded by a number of workers as an essential component of the sentinel node technique, being fundamental to achieving the highest possible sensitivity for detection of sentinel nodes in both melanoma and breast cancer. Reintgen and colleagues [8], Uren and co-workers [7, 9] and Pijpers and group [10] have all stressed the critical role of imaging in the successful identification of functional sentinel nodes in melanoma, this being due to its ability both to fully demonstrate lymphatic drainage patterns and to permit the accurate pre-operative localisation of all sentinel nodes visualised. Knowledge of these lymphatic drainage patterns has been found to predict difficulties in identifying the sentinel node and to assist in the prevention of false-negative biopsies in breast cancer by the incorrect interpretation of tracer uptake in multiple lymph nodes [11]. Statman and Guiliano cite their use of scintigraphy for selected inner quadrant breast tumours to establish the presence of drainage to the internal mammary node chain [12]; if this is seen they then perform interoperative lymphatic mapping to identify and biopsy the internal mammary sentinel node. Pre-operative marking of the location of the sentinel node can assist in guiding the site of incision for biopsy, and a number of standard techniques exist to facilitate accurate localisation of the sentinel node from the image data acquired. A clinical benefit to the patient then ensues, and it is stated that the efficiency of the technique is increased [13].

Scintigraphic visualisation of the sentinel node is technically straightforward and is a highly sensitive procedure if meticulous technique is observed. Specific guidelines are detailed later. The image data can be easily and relatively rapidly acquired. All lymph node basins under suspicion as potential pathways for drainage of the radiolabelled tracer from the primary tumour site may be investigated, thereby revealing the total population of functioning sentinel nodes. A sensitivity of 94% has been reported by Uren and co-workers in imaging 209 patients with melanoma [14]. Pijpers et al. reported the visualisation of sentinel nodes in all of 135 patients with melanoma [10], and Kapteijn et al. observed at least one sentinel node in 59 of 60 patients (98%) [15]. In their investigation of the sentinel node technique in breast cancer, Veronesi et al. [16] indicated successful identification of the sentinel node in 160 of 163 patients with breast cancer (98%) and Borgstein et al. reported that the sentinel node was successfully demonstrated in 116 of 130 patients (89%) [11].

Dynamic imaging also allows a more careful interpretation through study of the kinetics of the colloidal tracer immediately after administration, and this is particularly relevant in melanoma. It can readily demonstrate patterns of drainage, revealing pathways taken by the tracer in its migration from the injection site through the afferent lymphatic vessels to the true sentinel node(s), and has proven useful in eliminating the possible confusion caused by a second-echelon node concentrating tracer due to spillover from the true sentinel node, and located more closely to the primary tumour than the sentinel node [17].

A significant additional advantage of sentinel node imaging is its capability to demonstrate nodes potentially undetectable with the gamma detecting probe alone. This includes those sentinel nodes sited very close to, or actually underlying, the injection site [18], sentinel nodes located out of the expected lymph node basins and therefore beyond defined investigative boundaries for intra-operative probing, and finally those sentinel nodes situated very deep to the skin surface and/or demonstrating very low levels of tracer uptake.

The reproducibility of sentinel node imaging in melanoma has been shown to be acceptable. Uren and colleagues reported inter-observer agreement for 83 of the 84 (99%) node groups visualised in 51 patients [14]. The reproducibility between repeated scintigraphic studies has been investigated by Mudun and co-workers [6], who found agreement in 85% of 13 studies, and Kapteijn et al. [19], who reported agreement in 88% of 25 patients investigated.

Sentinel Node Imaging in Malignant Melanoma

Reintgen et al. have stated that sentinel node imaging acts as an indispensible "road map" for the sentinel node technique, and is required to identify all nodal basins at risk for metastatic disease, to identify both the location and the number of sentinel nodes, and to detect the presence of any in-transit nodes, where such nodes are considered to represent sentinel nodes in themselves [8]. Such in-transit nodes have been found to occur in 5% of patients studied [5]. Initial experience with the sentinel node technique in 82 patients with melanoma [20] revealed a 59% discordance between scintigraphic findings illustrating the drainage pathways for an intradermal administration of filtered ^{99m}Tc-sulphur colloid tracer

and classical anatomical patterns of lymphatic drainage for melanomas of the head, neck and trunk. The authors therefore recommend scintigraphy prior to biopsy or elective lymph node dissection for melanomas sited in these regions. Further experience over a number of studies has led to the recommendation that pre-operative scintigraphy be performed for all patients referred for sentinel node biopsy [21].

Uren and co-workers have also investigated the role of scintigraphy in melanoma in a number of studies using ^{99m}Tc-antimony sulphide colloid tracer injected intradermally; they encountered significant variability in lymphatic drainage between individuals [14] and a number of new and unexpected lymphatic drainage patterns contradicting classical anatomical theory [14, 22–25]. They report particular difficulties in the correct interpretation of lymph node drainage from the distal lower limb to multiple nodes in the groin, and advocate the need for early imaging to identify the first draining node(s) only as true sentinel nodes [7]. This finding is in agreement with that reported by Taylor et al. [17].

Pijpers and group performed dynamic imaging using intradermally administered technetium-99m colloidal albumin (nanocolloid). They reported that 39 of 41 patients (95%) demonstrated uptake of tracer into the sentinel node within 20 min of injection [13] and together with other workers define the first persisting focus of tracer accumulation to represent the true sentinel node, ignoring any later foci. Rapid tracer uptake and persisting retention are reported and are advocated as an advantageous feature of the particle size range for the colloidal albumin used [10]. Some spillover into satellite nodes is reported but is not felt to hinder correct interpretation when dynamic image data are available to assist in interpretation.

Sentinel Node Imaging in Breast Cancer

Veronesi and co-workers recently published a series of 163 patients with breast cancer to whom tracer was injected subdermally [16]. The kinetics for this route of administration are known to be more rapid, and the protocol included static imaging between 15 min and 3 h post-injection. The reported sensitivity in this study for detection of the sentinel node from scintigraphic data was 98% (160 of 163). It is reported that most sentinel nodes were visualised by 30 min, and always remained the hottest node thereafter.

The recently completed multicentre study co-ordinated by Krag et al. [18] reported a success rate for sentinel node detection of 93% (413/443 patients). It specified as its criterion for identification of the sentinel node that positive detection of a nodal hot spot must be made through the (un-marked) skin surface prior to surgical incision. By using gamma detecting probe-directed identification of the sentinel node at operation with no pre-operative imaging the surgeon is forced to survey the expected site "blind" and it may be postulated that the sensitivity of the technique is somewhat impaired by this stringent requirement. Pijpers et al. report that inclusion of sentinel node imaging identified a further 10% who may have failed to demonstrate a hot node at intra-operative probing [26], and this finding tends to support the above hypothesis. However, other recent large-scale patient studies performed by both Albertini et al. [27] and Cox et al. [28] using a combination of intra-operative lymphatic mapping and probe-guided biopsy, and by Guiliano et al. [29] using intra-operative lymphatic mapping alone, have not included sentinel node imaging in their published protocols.

Uren and co-workers have used sentinel node imaging to illustrate unexpected direct drainage to the supraclavicular or infraclavicular nodes in 20% of upper quadrant tumours from the circum-ferential peritumoral injection of ^{99m}Tc-antimony sulphide colloid tracer [30]. Internal mammary nodes were visualised in 12 of 34 patients (35%), and this finding certainly highlights the ability of a large field of view gamma camera to conveniently visualise all potential drainage paths in a single image. While a discussion of the role and signi-ficance of lymphatic drainage to the internal mammary node chain is beyond the scope of this chapter, it should be emphasised that Uren used a colloid with rather small particles for imaging.

The role of dynamic imaging in the sentinel node technique for breast cancer is presently un-defined and is probably an unnecessary addition to the imaging protocol. Pijpers et al. [26] chose not to perform dynamic imaging due to the slow kinetics of tracer flow expected from a peritumoral injection of ^{99m}Tc-colloidal albumin (nanocolloid). Their criteria for definition of a sentinel node as being the first nodal accumulation to reveal itself was modified to that of the node demonstrating the highest uptake at 2 h following administration, and it was shown by a larger subsequent study from the same group [11] that the predicted spill-over of tracer into a secondary satellite node is minimal and does not interfere with interpreta-tion. Borgstein et al. additionally reported that the primary usefulness of scintigraphic imaging may be in visualisation of the slow-phase kinetics of all those nodes bearing tracer, in an attempt to better interpret their relative rates of tracer clearance and in so doing reduce the false-negative rate of the technique to an acceptable level by identifying possible failures due to compromised lymphatic function [11].

Sentinel Node Imaging in Other Cancers

The success of the sentinel node technique in demonstrating the lymphatic drainage from the primary tumour in malignant melanoma has led to its direct extension to other cutaneous cancers – and in particular, neuroendocrine carcinoma of the skin (Merkel cell carcinoma), an aggressive cutaneous cancer with a natural history similar to melanoma. Using dynamic scintigraphic imag-ing and intra-operative gamma detection together with blue dye Javaheri et al. [31] reported suc-cessful detection of the sentinel node in one subject, and Ames and co-workers [32] success-fully located the sentinel node in all seven patients studied using intra-operative gamma detection only.

Following Cabanas' original exposition [33] of the sentinel node concept in penile carcinoma using lymphangiography, Kapteijn et al. [34] investigated 19 patients using a combination of dynamic lymphoscintigraphy, intra-operative gamma detection and blue dye. Ninety-one per-cent of observed sentinel nodes were detected intra-operatively. Inguinal lymph node dissection was performed only if the sentinel node was histologically positive for tumour, with one false-negative study reported – confirmed by the ap-pearance of an involved lymph node at follow-up 4 months later.

The sentinel node hypothesis has been investigated in vulval cancer by a number of groups. DeCesare and collagues [35] correctly identified the sentinel node in ten patients using a gamma detecting probe alone. De Hullu et al. [36] reported the successful detection of sentinel nodes in all ten patients studied using lymphoscintigraphy, intra-operative gamma detection and blue dye, and Terada et al. [37] found 100 % sensitivity for sentinel node detection in five patients also based upon a protocol incorporating all three approaches. De Cicco et al. [38] use dynamic lymphoscintigraphy and intra-operative detection to successfully identify the sentinel node in all of the 15 patients they investigated, reporting both a higher sensitivity and greater ease of detection technique than with sentinel node detection using blue dye alone [39], particularly for midline tumours.

The lymphatic drainage pattern of squamous cell carcinoma of the head and neck has also been investigated by imaging the flow of tracer. Koch et al. have detailed results from five patients with oral cancer, who received an intramucosal injection of tracer followed by dynamic lymphoscintigraphy and intra-operative gamma sentinel node detection [40]. Two cases were successfully investigated, but technical problems were encountered in detecting the sentinel node intra-operatively, in part due to their close physical proximity to the injection site. The effect of prior radiotherapy upon local lymphatic function, extrusion of tracer into the saliva and the inaccessibility of some primary tumour sites were also reported as significant impediments to the technique in this cancer.

Other applications have also been tried. Hosal and co-workers investigated patients receiving reconstruction with pectoralis major myocutaneous flaps after radical neck dissection for advanced cancer of the upper aerodigestive tract [41]. They used intradermally administered ^{99m}Tc-labelled dextran to image the pattern of lymphatic flow through both the neck and the pectoralis major myocutaneous flap with a further submucosal injection of ^{99m}Tc-sulphur colloid to localise the individual lymph nodes. Only when the flap was directly invaded by tumour, was there evidence of drainage to the internal mammary chain.

Sentinel Node Imaging Technique in Breast Cancer

Introduction

The following sections provide a detailed description of the sentinel node imaging protocol currently employed at our institution. It should be stated at the outset that this protocol is fundamentally directed at an (ongoing) investigative evaluation of the technique, and is accordingly specified to fulfil its requirements – in particular a dynamic imaging sequence is included to study the pharmacokinetics of the colloidal tracer. However, we believe that the guidelines provided constitute an aid to optimal sentinel node imaging in breast cancer, and many of the points discussed are equally relevant to achieving optimal images for the technique when applied to other cancers. Our practice has evolved, and has been further refined, over the course of the first 50 or so patients studied. We have modified and improved detailed aspects of the protocol in response to the technical problems encountered during initial studies, e.g. attenuation of the tracer due to overlying breast tissue and prevention of contamination, and when prompted by surgical and histopathological findings.

It is vital to note that the imaging protocol outlined here is optimised for the subdermal injection technique, and for the rapid kinetics to be expected from this route of administration of the chosen tracer. The protocol comprises three phases. The first is the initial rapid dynamic and static imaging sequence performed immediately after administration of tracer, with a second stage comprising a set of static images acquired at 2–4 h post-injection if the sentinel node should fail to appear scintigraphically within the time span of the first sequence. Should the sentinel node remain undetectable by imaging at this stage then we acquire a third sequence of static images at no less that 12 h after administration. For the majority of patients scheduled for operation the following day this last stage has proved a feasible proposition, but such images have limited diagnostic value and were acquired in the first 30 patients to establish that spillover of activity is negligible and that tracer is retained in the sentinel node. Our image data obtained at this stage have demonstrated that the sentinel node is both visible and should be detectable intra-operatively with a 10–15 MBq administration of a ^{99m}Tc-labelled colloid.

A single-headed gamma camera is certainly suitable for the acquisition of all sentinel node image data, although multi-detector systems can be equally adapted to perform the technique. We have used, and advocate, an appropriate high-resolution collimator (LEHR) to achieve maximal resolution of the lymphatic structures. It should also be stressed here that a gamma camera system with a large field of view (LFOV) detector – defined here as having a minimum dimension of 400 mm – is important to the success of the technique as it ensures full coverage of all those nodal basins likely to drain tracer from the injection site, together with appropriate local anatomical landmarks.

We strongly advocate the inclusion of relevant anatomical markers, e.g. for the nipple. These may be overlaid upon the image to indicate the location of the anatomical structure as an aid to the interpretation of scintigraphic findings. In particular we have found that transmission images acquired using a radioactive flood source are invaluable in localising the site of the detected sentinel node [42], and we have extended this technique to ensure optimal visualisation of both nodal uptake and body contours. The inclusion of anatomical information also has a valuable role in communicating findings to colleagues less familiar with the nature of sentinel node imaging. Flexible radioactive line sources outlining the anterior-posterior contour of the breast may also be of significant help in localising the sentinel node anatomically.

For scintigraphic findings to be interpreted successfully the patient must be positioned in a manner identical to that adopted for the surgical procedure. The projection of the site of the sentinel node upon the skin surface may be accurately marked by determining the location of tracer uptake with the aid of a radioactive point source and the gamma camera in the anterior oblique position. If this mark is subsequently confirmed with a gamma probe immediately after skin surface marking and is re-confirmed with the patient positioned at the time of surgery, it may then be used to plan the site of incision for sentinel node

biopsy with confidence. Other workers [9, 14] have also advocated that careful attention to technique is an especially important factor here.

Patient Preparation

The patient should be correctly positioned for imaging before the tracer is injected to ensure minimum delay between injection and start of the initial dynamic study. Patients undergoing excision of breast tumour with or without associated axillary node dissection will normally be placed supine with the arm on the affected side abducted at approximately 90°, and suitably supported (Fig. 1). A supine position also has the advantage here that it acts to reduce patient movement whilst image acquisition is in progress. In common with all radionuclide imaging procedures, the patient's bra and all relevant metallic items (coins, jewellery etc.) should be removed. Light clothing may be retained, but should not be such as to obstruct access for the injection and later skin surface marking. It should be established that the patient has not undergone a bone scan (or any other radionuclide study) in the 2 or, preferably, 3 days immediately preceding this investigation.

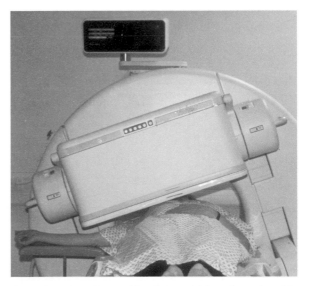

Fig. 1. Correct patient position for acquisition of anterior oblique views, demonstrating drainage of tracer from the breast to the axillary bed. Note that the entire breast, axilliary region and internal mammary chain are within the field of view of the detector

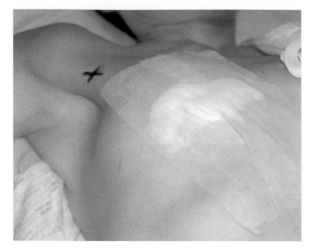

Fig. 2. Taping the breast onto the chest medially and inferiorly to prevent attenuation of any gamma rays emitted from the tracer in the axillary region. Any overlying breast tissue will attenuate gamma rays emitted from the tracer and will act to reduce the counts detected by the camera, imitating poor nodal uptake or, if attenuation is significant, a complete absence of migration of the tracer from the injection site

notch, extending to the supraclavicular fossa. The contours of the shoulder should also be included as a landmark for transmission imaging, if this is possible. For this reason the use of a gamma camera incorporating an LFOV detector is important to the success of the technique. If it is possible that the breast itself may overlie the injection site or nodal uptake within the axillary region, then the breast should be taped onto the chest medially and inferiorly such that it will not superimpose the sentinel node (Fig. 2) by overshadowing, or attenuating, the tracer with the overlying breast tissue.

Acquisition of Early Dynamic and Static Image Data

The patient is moved away from the detector and the tracer is injected as detailed in Chap. 5, with a note kept of the exact time of injection. The injection site itself is immediately sealed with a small adhesive plaster and massaged for 1 min by the patient. Immediately following this the patient is repositioned and dynamic imaging is commenced. Parameters for the acquisition of all image data are detailed in Table 1. Both the collimator and the pixel matrix should be chosen here to obtain the highest possible resolution for the images acquired.

Early images should be acquired in the relevant anterior oblique projection, with the detector orientated at approximately 30° anteriorly. The exact angle should be recorded and reproduced for all later acquisitions. It is important to ensure that the detector field of view covers the thorax from the midline to the lateral surface, and fully encloses the axillary region. The field of view should reach axially from the costal margin to the sternal

The dynamic sequence demonstrates the kinetics of tracer flow and highlights those afferent

Table 1. Parameters for acquisition of sentinel node image data

Collimator	Low energy high resolution (LEHR)
Pixel matrix: dynamic data	256 × 256 word depth, or highest available
Pixel matrix: static images	256 × 256 word depth
Pixel matrix: transmission image	256 × 256 word depth
Emission energy window	140 keV: 20% width; 3% offset or 15% width
Transmission energy window	^{57}Co: flood source 122 keV: 20% width ^{99m}Tc: flood source 140 keV: 20% width
Dynamic image projection	Anterior oblique
Static image projections	Matched anterior oblique and lateral
Transmission image projections	Matched anterior obliques and laterals
Imaging timepoints	Dynamic study from inj. to 45 min (90 × 10 s, 30 × 60 s) 5-minute static images at 45 min (mandatory) 5-minute static images at 2–4 h (mandatory if no visualisation before) 5- to 10-min static images at 12–24 h (optional)

lymphatic ducts directly draining the tracer – for a subdermal administration these may be most clearly observed in the early frames of the dynamic data sequence and for this reason image acquisition is commenced immediately after injection.

We have specified a high-resolution dynamic imaging protocol, collecting data into a 256 × 256 word mode (16 bit) pixel matrix with 10-s framing for 15 min, followed by 1-min framing for a further 30 min. This is optimised for the study of a collodal albumin tracer injected subdermally. Immediately following this a 5-min 256 × 256 word mode static image is acquired with the patient in the same position. This generates a static image of high technical quality approximately 45 min after the tracer is injected. By administering one subdermal injection of a small volume of tracer, we have not found it necessary to shield the injection site with a lead mask.

If the gamma camera has an electronic marking facility, i.e. not a radioactive marker, it is helpful to mark the position of the nipple on the static image (Figs. 3, 4). We have found that use of a radioactive point source marker can introduce unacceptable ambiguity when interpreting the image at a later stage, as the resulting detail may be easily confused with a site of genuine physiological tracer uptake if it is not meticulously documented.

A flexible, radioactive line source affixed to the skin is very helpful in delineating the anterior-posterior outline of the breast (Figs. 5, 6). This may be conveniently achieved using a commercially available cobalt-57-filled line source (or alternatively by the preparation of a thin-bore flexible tube filled with a solution of ^{99m}Tc and well sealed).

If the sentinel node is demonstrated at this stage, a 1- to 2-min 256 × 256 word mode transmission view is acquired with the patient remaining in the same position to assist in localising the sentinel node. This is achieved by placing a ^{57}Co or ^{99m}Tc flood source immediately beneath the patient, encompassing the field of view and orientated parallel to the camera face (Figs. 7, 8). An energy window appropriate to the flood source radionuclide is selected for the gamma camera and as such the image data obtained may contain in vivo count data primarily arising from radiation that has been scattered away from the sites of tracer uptake. For this reason the transmission

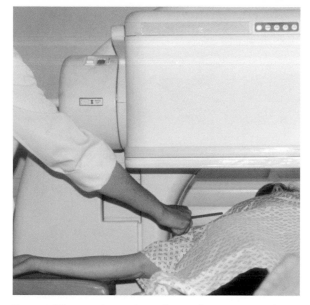

Fig. 3. Adding an electronic marker to the image. A radioactively tipped pencil marker containing a minute bead of ^{57}Co at its tip is used to identify the location of the nipple within the detector field of view. An arrow cursor is then manipulated on the computer display of this image field until it overlies the radioactive source. When accurate localisation is confirmed, a record of the position of the arrow cursor is confirmed for permanent attachment to the image file, allowing it to be displayed as a later optional overlay to the recorded image. The camera illustrated allows up to five such markers to be associated with each stored image. Note that the camera, patient and pencil source are widely separated for illustrative purposes

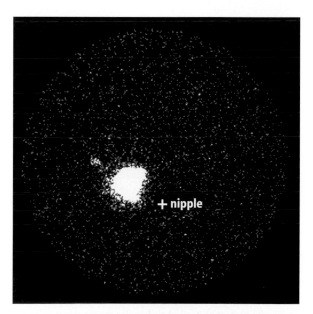

Fig. 4. A representative anterior oblique emission image with the electronic marker overlaid and anatomically annotated

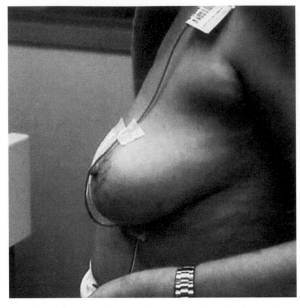

Fig. 5. Flexible marker source affixed to the skin. Sources are produced commercially containing ^{57}Co, a long-lived gamma emitter, sealed in a thin-bore flexible tube

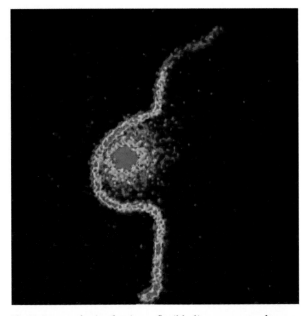

Fig. 6. Image obtained using a flexible line source to demonstrate the outline of the breast as an aid to anatomical localisation

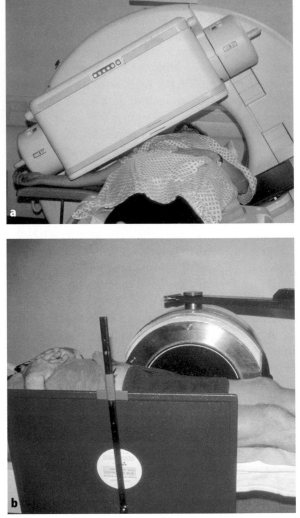

Fig. 7 a, b. Technique for acquisition of an anterior oblique transmission image (**a**), using a commercially produced "flood" source comprising a uniform distribution of the long half-life gamma emitting radionuclide ^{57}Co ($T_{1/2}$ 120 days, gamma energy 122 keV). Such sources are often used in gamma camera quality assurance programmes. By using a source holder, the radiation dose to the operator is reduced considerably (**b**)

image should not be used for diagnostic purposes but is acquired as a valuable tool for localising the sentinel node(s) anatomically. Careful technique should render the lung fields visible in the majority of patients.

Most gamma camera computer systems incorporate software permitting the operator to add together two count-normalised images. The maximum count density for the sentinel node in the emission image and the mean count density for a representative region of unattenuated transmission source are compared, weighted and used to add a weighted, count-normalised emission image to the associated transmission image, thereby generating an optimally "exposed" composite

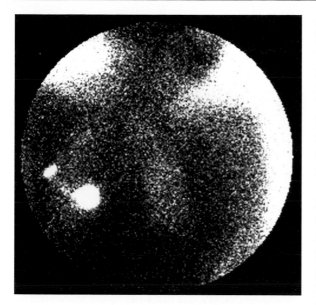

Fig. 8. A representative right anterior transmission image. The body outline is clearly seen, though a proportion of scattered radiation will always blur the exact boundary. The lung fields are often also visible due to the greater relative transmission of gamma rays through these low-density organs, and these act to provide a useful further anatomical landmark

image containing high-quality detail of the sentinel node(s) visualised. This technique also allows reduction of the time required to acquire the transmission data (Fig. 9). However, spatial registration of the two image sets is a prerequisite here, and is most simply achieved by ensuring that the patient is positioned identically for the acquisition of both sets of data and remains immobile throughout.

If by this stage one or more sentinel nodes are visualised, the position of each is now marked on the skin surface immediately overlying the site of tracer uptake. This assists in planning the incision for biopsy and is easily and accurately achieved by using a ^{57}Co point source marker and the gamma camera in persistence mode. The marker source is placed directly onto the skin surface and progressively advanced towards the site of tracer uptake until its own image superimposes upon that of the node. Once the exact site of uptake is located, the overlying skin is identified by accurate marking with a water-resistant permanent marker.

If the sentinel node is visualised at this stage, a lateral image is acquired to determine the depth of the node beneath the anterior skin surface. In upper outer quadrant lesions this image may

also reveal an undetected sentinel node if it has been obscured by activity from the injection site (Fig. 10). For optimal image quality the patient is positioned with the arm on the affected side overabducted until a comfortable position is found. This removes the arm as a source of attenuation between the sentinel node and the detector and minimises the distance between collimator face and source of activity, thereby improving image resolution (Fig. 11).

The detector field of view should extend from the cricoid to the costal margin. A 5-min 256 × 256 word mode static image is acquired in this position. Again, an electronic nipple marker may be included if the facility exists to store this. With the patient remaining in the same position, a 2-min transmission image is also acquired and processed as before.

Acquisition of Late Static Image Data

If no sentinel node is positively visualised at the initial stage, further data should be obtained between 2 and 4 h after injection. Anterior oblique and lateral static images are acquired as described for 5 min each, reproducing the previous positioning and imaging conditions. If a node is newly localised, then transmission image data are acquired for both anterior oblique and lateral images as described previously, together with a marker indicating the location of the nipple. Skin surface marking should also be performed as detailed above.

Acquisition of Delayed Static Image Data

If sentinel node localisation imaging remains negative and surgery is planned for the following day then further data can be acquired at approximately 18 – 24 h post-injection, and at not less than 12 h. The delayed image sequence should be acquired in an manner identical to early and late images, with corresponding transmission data if a sentinel node is positively visualised at this late stage. If a positive finding is indicated both the anterior oblique and lateral emission images should be acquired for 10 min to compensate for the loss of acquired counts through radioactive decay of the ^{99m}Tc-labelled tracer.

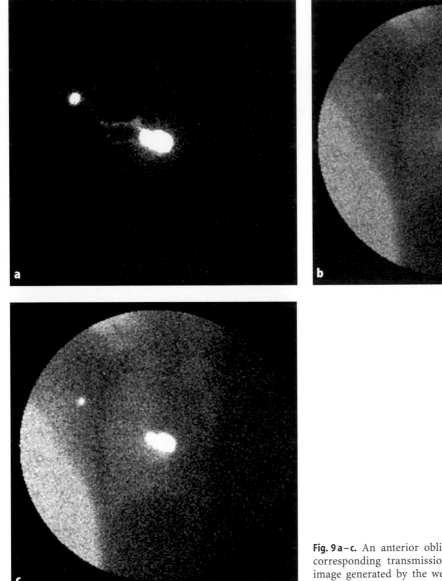

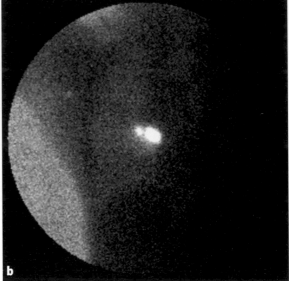

Fig. 9 a–c. An anterior oblique sentinel node image (a), its corresponding transmission image (b) and the combined image generated by the weighted addition of the two individual images (c)

Image Processing and Display

If acquired, the dynamic study should be initially reviewed in cine form to allow the underlying time-dependency of tracer uptake to be clearly visualised. Selected frames may then be extracted for individual display to best illustrate the migration of tracer, either as single frames or as the sum of a short sequence of consecutive frames. The entire dynamic sequence may be re-framed to display the acquired frames as a condensed sequence where each new frame now corresponds to a longer time interval, thereby reducing time resolution but increasing the visual quality of the frames that are generated.

Each static emission image is displayed alongside its corresponding combined emission and transmission image, with any anatomical landmarks superimposed, e.g. a marker for the nipple (see Fig. 4). Lateral images convey useful depth information and reveal hidden sentinel nodes. A comparison of equivalent anterior oblique and lateral images at differing timepoints will assist in the interpretation of tracer flow through the sentinel node(s).

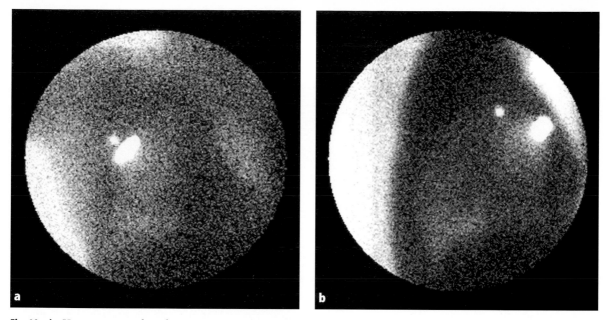

Fig. 10 a, b. Upper outer quadrant breast tumour with sentinel node almost obscured by overlying activity from the injection site in the anterior oblique image (**a**), but clearly visible beneath the injection site in the lateral image (**b**)

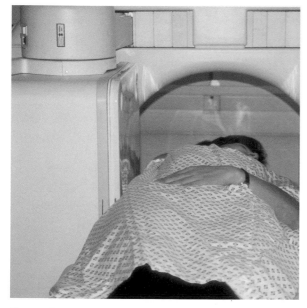

Fig. 11. Correct patient position for acquisition of a lateral image. Note that the entire thorax from the cricoid to the costal margin is within the field of view of the detector

Sentinel Node Imaging Technique in Melanoma

The merits of dynamic imaging in detecting the true sentinel node in malignant melanoma have already been mentioned, with many articles in the literature particularly attesting to the valuable information gained from the identification of un-expected drainage paths and an appreciation of the kinetics of lymphatic drainage from the injection site. We have successfully performed sentinel node imaging for melanoma, taking account of these observations and using a protocol based upon that detailed above for breast cancer.

For tumours in the distal lower limb brisk transport of tracer along the lymphatic vessels of the leg to the inguinal node basin is often observed. Tracking this rate of flow requires that dynamic imaging may need to be conducted in a sequence of uninterrupted stages as the camera is sequentially moved towards the torso. Late images may further assist in distinguishing between the true sentinel node and secondary, satellite nodes and in identifying in-transit nodes. Whole- or half-body scanned images are very useful in assimilating the drainage patterns established for truncal or lower limb lesions. Care should be taken to ensure that all possible drainage paths are imaged at this stage, using the dynamic data as a guide. Skin surface marking of all sentinel nodes is important, and as before, careful technique is vital to its accuracy. Anatomical marking and transmission imaging remain valuable components, and the transmission technique may be adapted for scan-

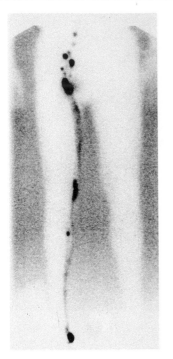

Fig. 12. Scanned transmission image of the passage of tracer from a melanoma located in the lower limb

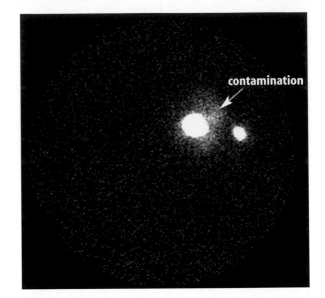

Fig. 13. Contamination of the injection site by spread of tracer. *Cause:* Tracer is absorbed onto the cotton wool swab used at injection, and is dispersed over the neighbouring skin during massage by the inappropriate further use of this swab. *Remedy:* Careful attention to injection technique (Chap. 5). The skin at the injection site should be immediately covered by a small adhesive plaster to prevent leakage of tracer from the puncture. The swab used at injection should be discarded immediately afterwards, and a new swab used to massage the skin

ned images by acquiring a second scan at a higher scan speed with the transmission source positioned on the lower detector head or suspended beneath the patient couch (Fig. 12).

Table 2 summarises key points relevant to clinical practice in respect of both melanomas and breast cancers.

Imaging Artefacts

Sentinel node imaging has few technical difficulties and potential pitfalls. However, as with all procedures, the potential for artefacts exist; many of these may be minimised by careful attention to the principles underlying good scintigraphic imaging technique and by following good radiation protection practice with regard to the prevention of contamination. Examples of specific representative artefacts are included here (Figs. 13–22), with an accompanying description of both their cause and some recommended strategies for prevention.

Table 2. Summary of key points for clinical practice

- Image the patient in the same position as at operation.
- Dynamic imaging is important in interpreting lymphatic drainage in melanoma.
- Marking the skin helps the surgeon to determine the site of incision.
- Imaging can display abnormal drainage patterns to unexpected lymph node basins and reduces the risk of false-negative cases.
- Imaging is an adjunct to lymphatic mapping and intra-operative detection for the successful localisation of sentinel nodes.
- Transmission imaging with a flood source is helpful for orientation and demonstrates anatomical landmarks.
- Use the camera's electronic marker facility to mark important anatomical landmarks, e.g. nipple.
- In upper outer quadrant carcinoma of the breast, retract the breast medially and downward to avoid overshadowing of the focal activity of the sentinel node by breast tissue.
- A lateral image is important for depth perception and in upper outer quadrant breast tumours helps to delineate the sentinel node if the injection site is close to the sentinel node.

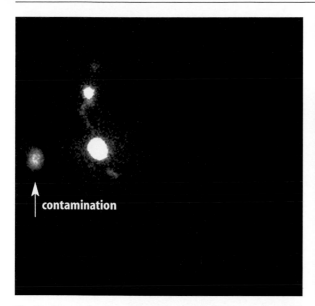

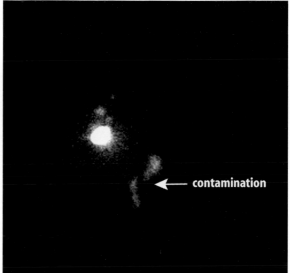

Fig. 14. Contamination of imaging couch due to a minor spill of tracer. *Cause:* The administered volume of tracer is very small, leading to a high activity concentration. One small drop of spilled solution is sufficient to significantly contaminate equipment, bedding or patient's clothing. *Remedy:* Careful attention to injection technique (Chap. 5). The tracer syringe should never be tapped to remove air bubbles, thereby causing aerosolisation of any radioactive tracer solution at the needle tip. Extreme care should be taken to avoid spilling any residual tracer solution whilst injecting, particularly onto the neighbouring skin. Any contaminated clothing or bedding should be immediately removed and replaced. An absorbent sheet should be used to cover the injection site (Chap. 5), incorporating a small aperture through which the injection(s) are administered

Fig. 15. Contamination of the patient's gown, due to a minor spill of tracer. *Cause:* A minor spill of tracer solution at injection, as in the previous example. *Remedy:* As for the previous example, careful attention to injection technique is critical to success (Chap. 5). All contaminated clothing or bedding should be immediately removed and replaced

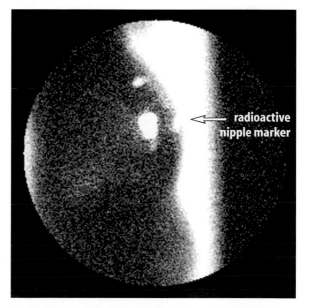

Fig. 16. Use of a radioactive nipple marker, without clear documentation as to its exact location. *Cause:* The image detail generated by using such a source is frequently indistinguishable in appearance from physiological tracer uptake and without unambigous documentation as to its site and form, use of radioactive markers may give rise to uncertainty when interpreting the image data. *Remedy:* Use the gamma camera's electronic anatomical marking facility if this is available

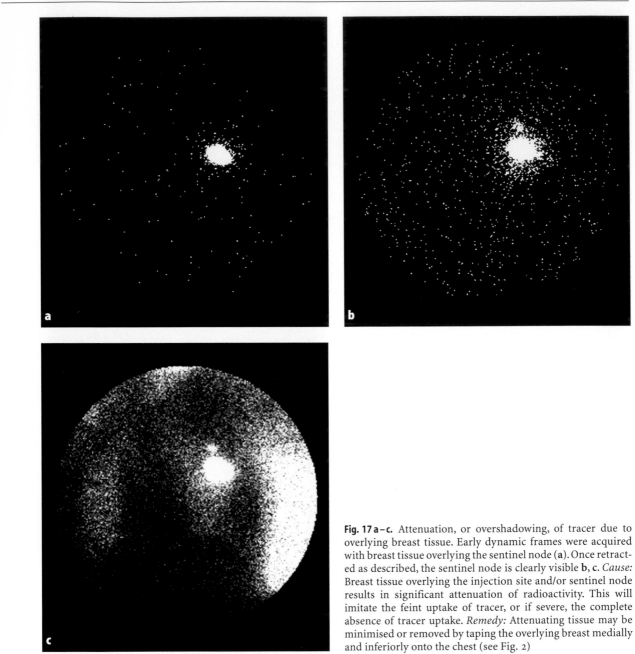

Fig. 17 a–c. Attenuation, or overshadowing, of tracer due to overlying breast tissue. Early dynamic frames were acquired with breast tissue overlying the sentinel node (**a**). Once retracted as described, the sentinel node is clearly visible **b**, **c**. *Cause:* Breast tissue overlying the injection site and/or sentinel node results in significant attenuation of radioactivity. This will imitate the feint uptake of tracer, or if severe, the complete absence of tracer uptake. *Remedy:* Attenuating tissue may be minimised or removed by taping the overlying breast medially and inferiorly onto the chest (see Fig. 2)

Fig. 20 a, b. Scattered radiation, from an injection site in the upper arm onto the metal base layer of an injection stand used to support the abducted arm. Scattered radiation, as seen in **a**, arises when gamma rays are scattered or deviated and are detected by the camera and assigned to an erroneous origin within the image. *Cause:* Gamma rays travelling inferiorly to the site shown here will pass through the intervening foam pad and will undergo a scattering interaction with the metal baseplate of the armrest (**b**). This may lead to some confusion in interpreting the image. *Remedy:* None. This physical phenomenon will occur if a site of significant tracer uptake lies close to a material of relatively high attenuating properties

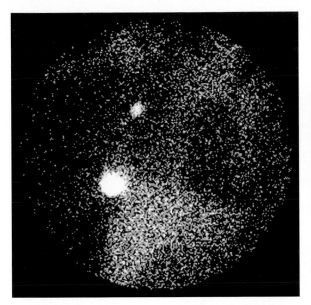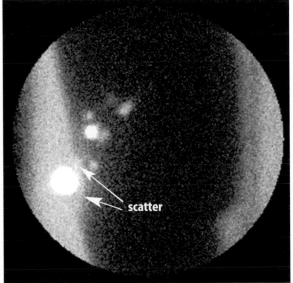

Fig. 18. Residual uptake of tracer due to an immediately preceding radionuclide scan. *Cause:* The patient had received a bone scan 2 days prior to the sentinel node procedure. For this investigation 800 MBq ⁹⁹ᵐTc-labelled phosphonate (HDP) was administered to the patient, in the prior knowledge of her breast cancer. Unusually, this patient also demonstrates some early hepatic uptake of the colloidal tracer due to its transport into the reticuloendothelial system. *Remedy:* Skeletal retention of phosphonate tracers in bone is normally significant, and therefore if at all possible a period of not less than 3 days should elapse before sentinel node mapping is performed to ensure that visualisation of the sentinel node is not confused with uptake of phosphonate tracer within the anterior ribs or sternum

Fig. 19. Scattered radiation, arising from the detection of gamma rays scattered or deviated by body tissue after their emission from the injection site with its very high concentration of tracer activity. *Cause:* Gamma rays emanate uniformly from the injection site in all directions. Those travelling posteriorly to the site shown here will pass through the intervening air gap and will undergo a scattering interaction with body soft tissues in the superficial skin layers of the pelvic area immediately posterior to the injection site. This may lead to an apparent, artefactual uptake in this region. *Remedy:* None. Whilst a rare occurrence in practice, this physical phenomenon will occur if a site of significant tracer uptake lies close to an intervening air gap. It may be identified as a possible cause by assessing the significance of the factors detailed here to the individual case considered

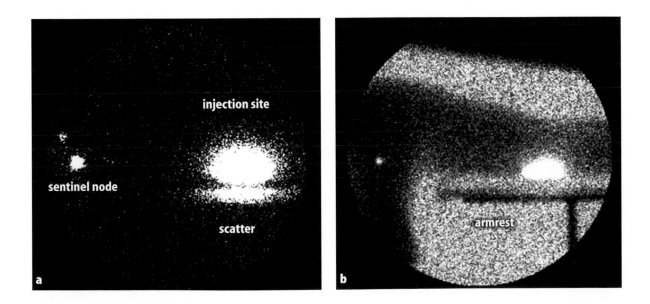

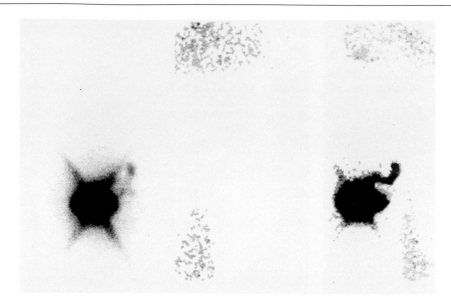

Fig. 21. Characteristic "starburst" artefact, allowing for confusion with the passage of tracer along a lymphatic tract. *Cause:* Gamma rays migrating from a high concentration of activity at the injection site will penetrate through the collimator at a glancing angle if either the design specification or the quality of construction of the collimator is suboptimal for the application. The honeycomb configuration of the lead collimator structure favours penetration of radiation through the hexagonal matrix of lead in the characteristic form of the starburst shown here. This source distribution may easily be confused with that arising from tracer uptake along one or more lymphatic tracts. *Remedy:* Use of a more highly specified collimator if this is possible; either rated as having higher resolution or, if absolutely necessary, as suitable for higher energy gamma emitters. Foil-fabricated collimator inserts are often more susceptible than those cast from lead in a single block

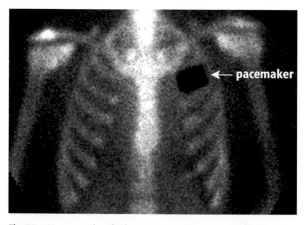

Fig. 22. An example of a bone scan with a pacemaker in situ. This problem may also occur with patients selected to receive sentinel node imaging. *Cause:* Metallic objects such as pacemakers will attenuate gamma rays. This phenomenon is very similar to the attenuation of X-rays through dense tissues and metallic objects within the body and will affect the images in a manner similar to that seen on radiographic images. *Remedy:* If suspected, the patient should be able to confirm the presence of a pacemaker in situ. A lateral view must then be obtained to exclude underlying tracer uptake

References

1. Morton DL, Wen DR, Wong JH, Economou JS, Cagle LA, Storm K, Foshag LJ, Cochran AJ. Technical details of intraoperative lymphatic mapping for early stage melanoma. *Arch Surg* 1992; 127:329–399
2. Alex JC, Krag DN. Gamma-probe guided localization of lymph nodes. *Surg Oncol* 1993; 2:137–143
3. Alex JC, Weaver DL, Fairbank JT, Rankin BS, Krag DN. Gamma-probe guided lymph node localization in malignant melanoma. *Surg Oncol* 1993; 2:303–308
4. Krag DN, Weaver DL, Alex JC, Fairbank JT. Surgical resection and radiolocalization of the sentinel node in breast cancer using a gamma probe. *Surg Oncol* 1993; 2:335–340
5. Albertini JJ, Cruse CW, Rapaport D, Wells K, Ross M, DeConti R, Berman CG, Jared K, Messina J, Lyman G, Glass F, Fenske N, Reintgen DS. Intraoperative radiolymphoscintigraphy improves sentinel node identification for patients with melanoma. *Ann Surg* 1996; 223:217–224
6. Mudun A, Murray DR, Herda SC, Eshima D, Shattuck LA, Vansant JP, Taylor AT, Alazraki NP. Early stage melanoma: lymphoscintigraphy, reproducibility of sentinel node detection, and effectiveness of the intraoperative gamma detecting probe. *Radiology* 1996; 199: 171–175

7. Uren RF, Howman-Giles R, Thompson JF, Shaw HM, Quinn MJ, O'Brien CJ, McCarthy WH. Lymphoscintigraphy to identify sentinel nodes in patients with melanoma. *Melanoma Res* 1994; 4:395–399

8. Reintgen D, Balch CM, Kirkwood J. Recent advances in the care of the patient with malignant melanoma. *Ann Surg* 1997; 225:1–14

9. McCarthy WH, Thompson JF, Uren RF. Invited commentary. Minimal access surgery for staging of malignant melanoma. *Arch Surg* 1995; 130:659–660

10. Pijpers R, Borgstein PJ, Meijer S, Hoekstra OS, van Hattum LH, Teule GJJ. Sentinel node biopsy in melanoma patients: dynamic lymphoscintigraphy followed by intraoperative gamma probe and vital dye guidance. *World J Surg* 1997; 788–793

11. Borgstein PJ, Pijpers R, Comans EF, van Diest PJ, Boom RP, Meijer S. Sentinel node biopsy in breast cancer: guidelines and pitfalls of lymphoscintigraphy and gamma probe detection. *J Am Coll Surg* 1998; 186:275–283

12. Statman R, Guiliano AE. The role of the sentinel node in the management of patients with breast cancer. *Adv Surg* 1996; 30:209–221

13. Pijpers R, Collet GJ, Meijer S, Hoekstra OS. The impact of dynamic scintigraphy and gamma probe guidance on sentinel node biopsy in melanoma. *Eur J Nucl Med* 1995; 22:1238–1241

14. Uren RF, Howman-Giles RB, Shaw HM, Thompson JF, McCarthy WH. Lymphoscintigraphy in high-risk melanoma of the trunk; predicting draining node groups, defining lymphatic channels and locating the sentinel node. *J Nucl Med* 1993; 34:1435–1440

15. Kapteijn BAE, Nieweg OE, Muller SH, Liem IH, Hoefnagel CA, Rutgers EJTh, Kroon BBR. Validation of gamma probe detection of the sentinel node in melanoma. *J Nucl Med* 1997; 38:362–366

16. Veronesi U, Paganelli G, Galimberti V, Viale G, Zurrida S, Bedoni M, Costa A, deCicco C, Geraghty JG, Luini A, Sacchini V, Veronesi P. Sentinel node biopsy to avoid axillary dissection in breast cancer with clinically negative lymph nodes. *Lancet* 1997; 349:1864–1867

17. Taylor A, Murray D, Herda S, Vansant J, Alazraki NP. Dynamic scintigraphy to identify the sentinel and satellite nodes. *Clin Nucl Med* 1996; 10:755–758

18. Krag D, Weaver D, Ashikaga T, Moffat F, Klimberg VS, Shriver C, Feldman S, Kusminsky R, Gadd M, Kuhn J, Harlow S, Beitsch P. The sentinel node in breast cancer – a multicenter validation study. *N Engl J Med* 1998; 339:941–946

19. Kapteijn BAE, Nieweg OE, Valdés-Olmos RA, Liem IH, Baidjnath Panday RKL, Hoefnagel CA, Kroon BBR. Reproducibility of lymphoscintigraphy for lymphatic mapping in cutaneous melanoma. *J Nucl Med* 1996; 37:972–975

20. Norman J, Cruse CW, Espinosa C, Cox C, Berman C, Clark AR, Saba H, Wells K, Reintgen D. Redefinition of cutaneous lymphatic drainage with the use of lymphoscintigraphy for malignant melanoma. *Am J Surg* 1991; 162:432–437

21. Reintgen D. More rational and conservative surgical strategies for malignant melanoma using lymphatic mapping and sentinel node biopsy techniques. *Curr Opin Oncol* 1996; 8:152–158

22. Uren RF, Howman-Giles RB, Thompson JF, Shaw HM, McCarthy WH. Lymphatic drainage from peri-umbilical skin to internal mammary nodes. *Clin Nucl Med* 1995; 20:254–255

23. Uren FR, Howman-Giles RB, Thompson JF, Quinn MJ, O'Brien C, Shaw HM, Bosch CMJ, McCarthy WH. Lymphatic drainage to triangular intermuscular space lymph nodes in melanoma on the back. *J Nucl Med* 1996; 37:964–966

24. Uren RF, Howman-Giles R, Thompson JF, Quinn MJ. Direct lymphatic drainage from the skin of the forearm to a supraclavicular node. *Clin Nucl Med* 1996; 21:387–389

25. Uren RF, Howman-Giles R, Thompson JF, McCarthy WH. Exclusive lymphatic drainage from a melanoma on the back to intraabdominal lymph nodes. *Clin Nucl Med* 1998; 23:71–73

26. Pijpers R, Meijer S, Hoekstra OS, Collet GJ, Comans EFI, Boom RPA, van Diest PJ, Teule GJJ. Impact of lymphoscintigraphy on sentinel node identification with technetium-99m-colloidal albumin in breast cancer. *J Nucl Med* 1997; 38:366–368

27. Albertini JJ, Lyman GH, Cox C, Yeatman T, Bladucci L, Ku N, Shivers S, Berman C, Wells K, Rapaport D, Shons A, Horton J, Greenberg H, Nicosia S, Clark R, Cantor A, Reintgen DS. Lymphatic mapping and sentinel node biopsy in the patient with breast cancer. *JAMA* 1996; 276:1818–1822

28. Cox C, Pendas S, Cox JM, Joseph E, Shons AR, Yeatman T, Ku NN, Lyman GH, Berman C, Haddad F, Reintgen DS. Guidelines for sentinel node biopsy and lymphatic mapping of patients with breast cancer. *Ann Surg* 1998; 227:645–653

29. Guiliano AE, Dale PS, Turner RR, Morton DL, Evans SW, Krasne DL. Improved axillary staging of breast cancer with sentinel lymphadenectomy. *Ann Surg* 1995; 222:394–401

30. Uren RF, Howman-Giles RB, Thompson JF, Malouf D, Ramsey-Stewart G, Niesche FW, Renwick SB. Mammary lymphoscintigraphy in breast cancer. *J Nucl Med* 1995; 36:1775–1780

31. Javaheri S, Cruse CW, Stadelmann WK, Reintgen DS. Sentinel node excision for the diagnosis of metastatic neuroendocrine carcinoma of the skin: a case report. *Ann Plast Surg* 1997; 39:299–302

32. Ames SE, Krag DN, Brady MS. Radiolocalization of the sentinel node in Merkel cell carcinoma: a clinical analysis of seven cases. *J Surg Oncol* 1998; 67:251–254

33. Cabanas RM. An approach for the treatment of penile carcinoma. *Cancer* 1977; 39:456–466

34. Kapteijn BAE, Horenblas S, Nieweg OE, Meinhardt W, Hoefnagel CA, De Jong D, Kroon BBR. Dynamic sentinel node procedure in penile cancer: a report on 19 cases. In: Kapteijn BAE. *Biopsy of the sentinel node in melanoma, penile carcinoma and breast carcinoma – the case for lymphatic mapping.* Academisch Proefschrift, Universiteit van Amsterdam, 1997

35. DeCesare SL, Fiorica JV, Roberts WS, Reintgen D, Arango H, Hoffman MS, Puleo C, Cavanagh D. A pilot study utilizing intraoperative lymphoscintigraphy for identification of the sentinel nodes in vulvar cancer. *Gynecol Oncol* 1977; 66:425–428

36. De Hullu JA, Doting E, Piers DA, Hollema H, Aalders JG, Schraffordt Koops H, Boonstra H, von der Zee AGJ. Sentinel node identification with technetium-99m-labelled nanocolloid in squamous cell cancer of the vulva. *J Nucl Med* 1998; 39:1381–1385

37. Terada KY, Coel MN, Ko P, Wong JH. Combined use of intraoperative lymphatic mapping and lymphoscintigra-

phy in the management of squamous cell cancer of the vulva. *Gynecol Oncol* 1998; 70:65–69

38. De Cicco C, Sideri M, Bartolomei M, Maggioni A, Columbo N, Bocciolone L, Chinol M, Leonardi L, Mangioni C, Paganelli G. Sentinel node detection by lymphoscintigraphy and gamma detecting probe in patients with vulvar cancer. *J Nucl Med* 1997; 38(5):33P

39. Levenback C, Burke TW, Gershenson DM, Morris M, Malpica A, Ross MI. Intraoperative lymphatic mapping for vulvar cancer. *Obstet Gynecol* 1994; 84:163–167

40. Koch WM, Choti MA, Civelek AC, Eisele DW, Saunders JR. Gamma probe-directed biopsy of the sentinel node in oral squamous cell carcinoma. *Arch Otolaryngol Head Neck Surg* 1998; 124:455–459

41. Hosal N, Turan E, Aras T. Lymphoscintigraphy in pectoralis major myocutaneous flaps. *Arch Otolaryngol Head Neck Surg* 1994; 120:659–661

42. West JH, Seymour JC, Drane WE. Combined transmission-emission imaging in lymphoscintigraphy. *Clin Nucl Med* 1993; 18:762–764

CHAPTER 7

Surgical Techniques

Introduction

With the sentinel node technique gaining popularity as an important and minimally invasive staging procedure in surgical oncology, there is renewed interest in the structure and function of the lymphatic system. The lymph nodes are highly specialised immunocompetent organs which are located along the length of lymphatic vessels [1]. Each lymph node is covered by a capsule of dense connective tissue that extends strands called trabeculae into the node, dividing it into several compartments. Within the lymph node parenchyma there are two main regions: cortex and medulla. The outer cortex contains many lymphoid follicles, which are regions of densely packed lymphocytes. T lymphocytes and macrophages and follicular dendritic cells which participate in the activation of T cells are located on the outer rim of these lymphoid follicles. The germinal centre is the lighter staining central area of a follicle where B lymphocytes proliferate into antibody-secreting plasma cells [2]. The inner region of a lymph node is the medulla. Here lymphocytes are tightly packed in strands called medullary cords. Lymph flows through a node in one direction. It enters through the afferent lymphatic vessels, which penetrate the convex surface of the node at several points [2].

Lymph enters the subcapsular sinus and then through cortical and medullary sinuses exits the lymph node via one or two wider efferent lymphatic vessels. These lymphatic sinuses contain numerous macrophages [1]. The lymph node filters foreign substances which can be trapped by the reticular fibres within the node. Macrophages may destroy these by phagocytosis and lymphocytes also play a role in the immunological response. In the sentinel node context the colloidal particles and the blue dye are taken up by macrophages; this point is illustrated in Chap. 10 and in Chap. 11, case no. 16.

Sentinel Node Detection in Breast Cancer

The surgical techniques used in the intra-operative detection of the sentinel node have varied significantly, ranging from blue dye lymphatic mapping alone to probe-guided surgery alone or in combination with the blue dye technique. Giuliano et al. [3] performed lymphatic mapping by using isosulfan blue vital dye, which was injected in a peritumoral fashion into the breast parenchyma in 174 patients. A success rate of 65% and a sensitivity of 75% were reported, although higher success rates were subsequently achieved with experience. In a pilot study performed by Krag and associates [4] the technique of probe-guided localisation of the radiolabelled sentinel node was introduced after their initial success in staging patients with melanoma [5, 6]. The success rate of this technique was 82%, with a predictive accuracy of 100%. In a study performed by Albertini and associates [7], combining the blue dye technique and probe-guided surgery in 62 patients, a success rate of 92% was reported, with 100% accuracy in predicting the axillary node status. These authors concluded that the addition of the gamma detection probe increased the success rate from 73% to 92%, as in 12 patients blue dye did not appear in the lymph nodes but focal hot spots were detected by the probe. A higher detection rate of 98% was reported by Veronesi and co-workers [8], with a false-negative rate of 5.4%, after subdermal injection of colloidal albumin and probe-guided surgery.

Blue Dye Lymphatic Mapping

With the intraparenchymal injection of the blue dye alone, the success rate for identification of the sentinel node varies between 65% and 93%, with a reported false-negative rate of 0%–12% [9, 10]. The lymphatic mapping technique with blue dye can be tedious and a significant training element is involved [11]. The extent of the dissection and disruption of lymphatic channels can be higher as compared with probe-guided surgery; moreover, localisation of sentinel nodes in lymphatic basins other than the axillary basin is not possible [12–14].

Timing of injection of the blue dye is crucial for the success of the procedure. If it is injected too early, there would be extensive blue staining of lymph nodes in the nodal basin, making the task of sentinel node localisation impossible. On the other hand if the injection is administered too late, successful localisation may fail owing to the inability of the dye to reach the sentinel node because of inadvertent disruption of the lymphatic channels during dissection. It seems that the optimal time for injection of the blue dye is approximately 5 min prior to the surgical incision, and we have had satisfactory results in this way.

The reported side-effects associated with the patent blue dye include cutaneous rash, observed in particular in patients with a previous history of allergic reaction. Blue to green discoloration of urine (Fig. 1) can be a cause for concern to the patient postoperatively, and this effect needs to be explained to the patient. Persistence of blue stain after intradermal injection of the patent blue dye

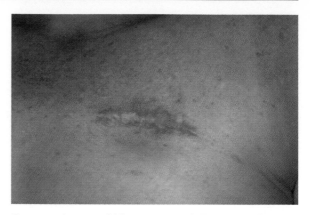

Fig. 2. Persistence of blue staining of skin 6 months postoperatively

can happen [15], and patients need to be warned about this. In most cases this gradually disappears with time but occasionally it leads to permanent tattooing of the skin (Fig. 2).

Rodier and Janser report an anaphylactic reaction as a result of administration of the patent blue dye in one patient in a study of 65 patients [15].

Probe-Guided Surgery

The success rate of gamma detection probe-guided surgery is superior to that of blue dye mapping alone [7, 8, 16]. As already mentioned, the experience of Albertini et al. [7] indicates that the addition of a gamma detection probe increases the success rate of sentinel node localisation from 73% to 92%.

Knowledge of the location of the sentinel node before surgical exposure is what differentiates probe-guided surgery and lymphatic mapping [5, 17, 18]. The site of the sentinel node is identified even before the incision is made. Another important advantage of probe-guided surgery is that complete excision of the sentinel nodes can be verified by directing the probe into the wound to measure the residual activity.

Various reports suggest that combination of blue dye lymphatic mapping and probe-guided sentinel node localisation is advantageous [7, 16, 19, 20]. The overall success of sentinel node localisation is maximised and the incidence of false-negative results reduced when both techniques are used in conjunction. This is because a probe will give

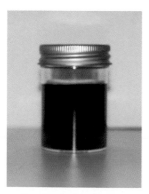

Fig. 1. Dark blue discoloration of urine due to patent blue dye injection, 18 h postoperatively

the surgeon a sense of direction and allows detection of non-visible nodes due to their radioactive content, whilst the blue dye helps as a visual guide when the node is exposed. Combination of the two techniques may also accelerate the learning curve of each method used in isolation. It has also been our experience that additional information from pre-operative lymphoscintigraphy is very helpful in predicting the success of sentinel node biopsy.

Intra-operative Sentinel Node Detection Technique

It is important to make sure that the gamma detector probe is in good working condition before use; in particular, if the detector is battery operated one must ensure that it is properly charged. Failure of sentinel node localisation has been reported as a result of technical malfunction of the gamma detection probe [19]. In collaboration with the physicist a regular sensitivity test of the probe is highly recommended to safeguard against the undetected gradual degradation of sensitivity over time. This is facilitated by using standard sources like iodine-129 or cobalt-57 in a reproducible fashion for the regular measurement of sensitivity (Fig. 3).

The characteristics of the gamma detector probes and electromedical safety issues are described in Chap. 3. The surgeon needs to be familiar with the function of the probe that is used. Once the patient has been anaesthetised and prepared for the operative procedure, the probe and its cable are

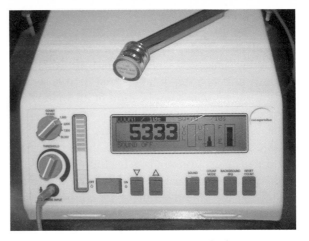

Fig. 3. Gamma detection probe with a standard source

covered with suitable sterile plastic tubing; for extra safety, to avoid contamination the probe can be inserted in a sterile glove before covering it with plastic tubing. The probe's display unit is placed in front of the surgeon. It is good clinical practice to ensure that the probe is well secured during operation to avoid its accidental fall during surgery (Fig. 4). Probes are very sensitive to damage and costly to replace and care needs to be taken to safeguard against such an accident.

Fig. 4. a Theatre set up. The probe's display unit is facing the surgeon. **b** Probe properly secured during surgery

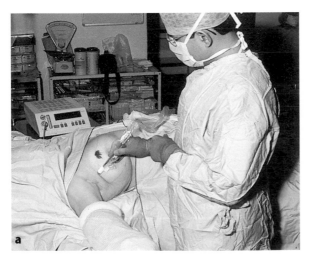

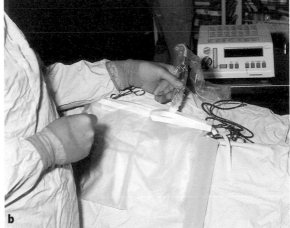

Injection of Patent Blue Dye

It is good practice to inform the anaesthetist about the patent blue dye injection, as occasionally total body blue coloration is noted, and this may cause confusion with hypercapnia or pulmonary embolism [15]. The complication of an anaphylactic reaction as a result of blue dye administration must be considered [15]. We inject 1.5–2 ml of patent blue dye subdermally into the skin overlying the primary tumour. It is best to use a syringe with a Luer lock, which avoids any accidental spillage of the blue dye during its administration under pressure. To avoid spillage of the dye, it is important to ensure that the syringe is empty before it is withdrawn or, if this is not possible, to avoid any pressure on the plunger during withdrawal. The injection site is gently massaged. In non-palpable breast carcinoma the injection site can be marked under image guidance before surgery or, if the lesion is localised by a wire, the wire can be used as a guide to the administration of the blue dye. Before the incision is made all the blue-stained swabs are removed from the operation field and if the gloves are stained, these are changed. This is to avoid any confusion as a result of inadvertent staining of axillary tissue during dissection. Figure 5 demonstrates that the lymphatic duct can be visualised through the intact skin as a blue line after patent blue dye injection and that this corresponds to the lymphatic trunk seen on the dynamic image.

Determination of the Site of Incision

It has been our observation that whilst the skin marking done under the gamma camera is helpful, it is not always accurate, as this is performed only in one plane. It is important to verify the location of the sentinel node before the incision is made. We apply the probe (Neoprobe 1500) over the axilla around the skin mark and, by slow movement of the probe over the skin, locate the centre of the hot spot which has maximum activity. This is confirmed by high-pitch audio signals from the probe and a high radiation count as compared with the background activity (Fig. 6).

Measurement of the Background Activity

Background radiation activity is measured by pointing the probe away from the injection site.

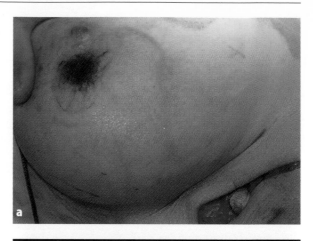

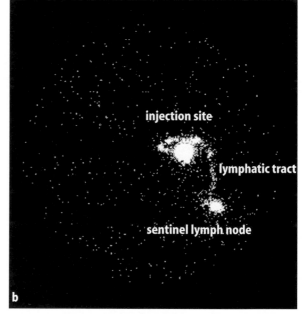

Fig. 5. **a** A blue lymphatic tract after patent blue dye injection. **b** The dynamic image sequence on the same patient

In most cases we perform this by applying the probe around the sternal notch area and making sure that it is held at a 90° angle to the body (Fig. 7).

Establishment of the "Line-of-sight"

Establishing the "line-of-sight" is one of the important advantages of probe-guided surgery, as it gives the surgeon a sense of direction (the term used by Krag and associates). In this way the dissection is not blind and the surgeon determines the shortest route to the sentinel node by changing the angle of the probe's tip. As a result tissue disruption is minimal. It is important to avoid pointing the probe towards the injection site as this will artificially

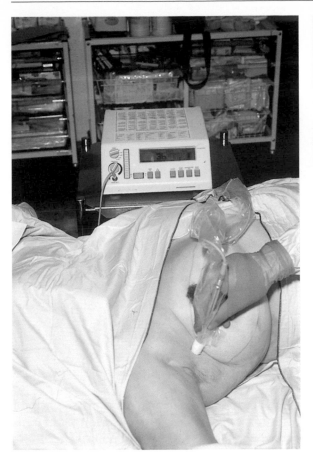

Fig. 6. Detection of the sentinel node site through the skin using the Neoprobe 1500

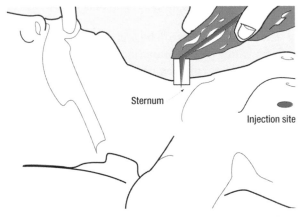

Fig. 7. Recording of background activity

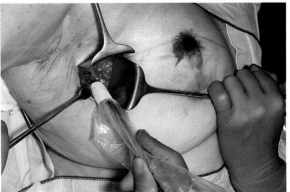

Fig. 8. Combination of probe and blue-dye detection of the sentinel node

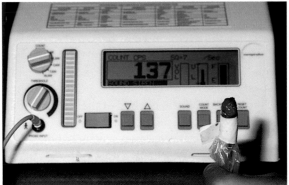

Fig. 9. Ex vivo activity count

raise the radiation count. The audio signal's pitch increases as the sentinel node is approached and this helps the surgeon to accurately locate the hot spot without needing to survey the control unit (Fig. 8).

Excision of the Sentinel Node

The sentinel node is approached by a blunt dissection with special attention to haemostasis. The line-of-sight is established soon after the incision. The direction of dissection is constantly checked with the probe. If a blue-stained lymphatic duct is encountered during dissection, care is taken not to transect it as this will lead to leakage of the blue dye and blue discoloration of the axillary tissue [15].

After the sentinel node has been localised by the probe, additional visual assistance from the blue dye can also help, and the radioactivity of the node is recorded by the probe as "in vivo counts/s". The radioactive node is excised and the "ex vivo" count is measured. To avoid any interference from the background radioactivity of surrounding areas, the ex vivo count is best done by applying the node onto the probe. Pointing upwards (Fig. 9).

The sentinel node is labelled separately and sent fresh to the laboratory for further analysis. As we are assessing the role of imprint cytology in the intra-operative diagnosis of the sentinel node, the node is bi-valved in the operating theatre and imprint cytology is obtained as described in detail in Chap. 10.

Verification of Sentinel Node Excision

It is very important to confirm the complete removal of the radioactive nodes. This is achieved by re-applying the probe into the wound. A careful measurement of the residual activity is done. It is important to angle the probe in all directions to ensure that there is no residual sentinel node. This is one of the clear advantages of radiocolloid-guided surgery. It has been our observation that the probe usually detects slightly higher radiation count than the background and we feel that this is probably due to the activity from the transected lymphatic ducts (Fig. 10). Krag and associates advocate removal of radioactive nodes until the background activity at the bed of the sentinel node resection site is reduced to less than 10 % of that of the most radioactive resected sentinel node.

Completion Lymphadenectomy

After the sentinel node has been excised, the standard axillary node dissection is performed. This is because we are at present still validating the predictive value of sentinel node biopsy in determining the status of the axillary lymphatic basin.

Fig. 10. a Residual activity measurement after excision of the sentinel node. **b** The probe is applied in all directions

Pitfalls

Upper Outer Quadrant Lesions

Upper outer quadrant lesions can pose some difficulty during gamma probe localisation [27]. This is due to the close proximity of the injection site to the sentinel node, which causes radiation scattered from the injection site to reach the detector. This is termed the shine-through phenomenon. In a multicentre validation study by Krag et al. [12], all false-negative results occurred in patients who had a primary carcinoma in the lateral half of the breast. To overcome this problem, the following manoeuvres might prove helpful:

1. Angling of the probe away from the injection site.
2. Use of additional collimation to reduce the scattered radiation and background activity.
3. Sometimes use of a "blocking plate" made of steel or tungsten can be of value to shield the injection site and reduce the interference from the injection site.
4. In exceptional circumstances it may be helpful to excise the primary lesion prior to the sentinel node biopsy in order to remove the strong source of radioactivity from the proximity of the sentinel node.

Reduced Functional Capacity of the Sentinel Node

■ **Extensive Infiltration by Metastatic Carcinoma.** Preservation of the functional capacity of the lymph node, permitting nodal uptake of the radioactive colloid, is critical for successful localisation

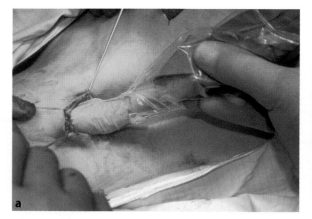
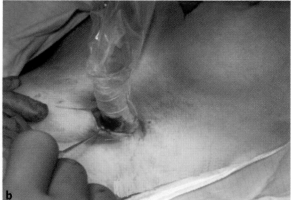

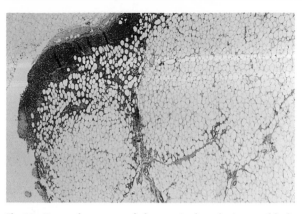

Fig. 11. Fat replacement of the sentinel node in an elderly patient

[16]. Nodal uptake is progressively reduced if there is excessive infiltration with metastatic carcinoma. This is a cause for concern as it can lead to a false-negative sentinel node biopsy. The problem of reduced functional capacity of the lymph node is also described by Borgstein et al. as one of the potential pitfalls [16]. In two of four patients in their study the less radioactive non-sentinel node contained excessive tumour infiltration as compared with hot sentinel nodes which were not involved with carcinoma. Borgstein et al. recommend careful scrutiny of the lymphoscintigraphic images to overcome this potential pitfall. We have observed this phenomenon in our study, as shown in Chapt. 11, case no. 14.

■ **Fatty Degeneration of the Sentinel Node.** The other reason for reduced functional capacity of lymph node is fatty degeneration of the axillary lymph node. We have observed this condition in elderly patients (Fig. 11). Tracer uptake by the lymph node is reduced, which in turn makes the probe localisation difficult. Additionally, it may pose difficulty in preparing frozen sections for histological analysis. Additional use of blue dye and careful interpretation of lymphoscintigraphic scans may help to overcome this problem.

Internal Mammary Nodes

There are no clear guidelines regarding the issue of internal mammary node dissection. It is our policy not to biopsy these nodes although others ad-

vocate their routine excision [21]. Moreover the detection rate of internal mammary nodes varies significantly between groups. Other variables seem to affect the detection rate of internal mammary nodes, and amongst these the particle size and the injection technique appear to be the two most important. We hope that the ongoing large multi-centre trials will resolve this issue.

Sentinel Node Detection in Malignant Melanoma

Sentinel node detection in malignant melanoma is discussed in detail in Chap. 12. The sentinel node concept was first introduced by Morton et al. [18], who performed lymphatic mapping and sentinel node biopsy using vital blue dye. There are inherent limitations associated with the use of blue dye only, including:

1. A lower rate of detection of the sentinel node
2. Inability to localise the sentinel node pre-operatively
3. Inability to locate unusual lymphatic basins
4. The requirement for more extensive surgery, as a skin flap must be raised to follow the blue lymphatic tract
5. Impossibility of performing the procedure under local anaesthesia
6. A more extensive learning curve

Significant progress has been achieved with introduction of probe-guided surgery. In a study performed by Alex and Krag [5] the following key advantages over blue lymphatic mapping were seen:

1. Precise localisation of the sentinel node on the skin surface
2. Constant guidance of the surgeon intra-operatively
3. Identification of in-transit nodes
4. Verification that the correct node has been biopsied
5. Determination of the possible presence of residual lymph nodes
6. Operation with a smaller incision and under local anaesthetic, as a day case

As in breast cancer, blue dye lymphatic mapping and the gamma detection probe technique are complementary, since use of blue dye provides additional information relevant to the distinction between a sentinel node and a second-echelon node [22] (Fig. 12).

Intra-operative Detection Technique

In our study every patient has undergone pre-operative dynamic and static lymphoscintigraphy, and the lymphatic basin and the sentinel node(s) have been identified pre-operatively.

The lymphatic basin is prepared in standard fashion and 1.5 – 2 ml of patent blue dye is injected subdermally around the lesion or on either side of the previous biopsy scar (Fig. 12). The gamma detection probe in a sterile plastic sleeve is used to verify the location of the sentinel node, and the site of incision is determined. The probe can constantly guide the surgeon to the sentinel node and the blue dye helps to locate the node more easily (Fig. 13).

In a study performed by Pijpers et al. [24], evaluating 135 patients with malignant melanoma, it was concluded that the key to success of sentinel node detection lies in combining dynamic lymphoscintigraphy with subsequent intra-operative gamma probe and blue dye guidance. After the sentinel node has been excised, the probe is re-applied to the wound to check the radioactivity and ensure that there is no residual sentinel node.

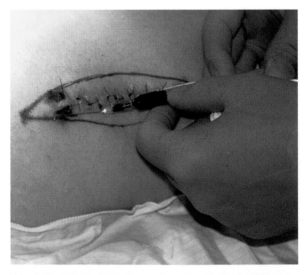

Fig. 12. Injection of patent blue dye on either side of the previous biopsy scar

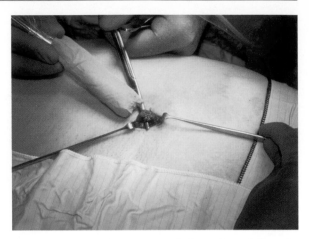

Fig. 13. Sentinel node detection with the probe and dye techniques combined

This is one of the greatest advantages of probe-guided surgery. The ex vivo count of the sentinel node is recorded and the node is processed as explained earlier.

Sentinel Node Detection in Penile Cancer

The sentinel node concept was first described by Cabanas [23] in the staging of penile carcinoma. He proposed this concept after an 8-year study of lymphangiograms, anatomical dissections and microscopic reports of 100 patients, including 80 with penile carcinoma, ten with inflammatory diseases of the penis and ten normal volunteers.

Intra-operative Detection Technique

In principle, the sentinel biopsy technique in penile carcinoma is no different form that in breast cancer and melanoma, described above. Pre-operative imaging is very helpful in delineating the lymphatic basin and the sentinel node in the groin. The use of patent blue dye is a useful adjunct to probe-guided surgery. The blue dye is injected around the tumour and the sentinel node is localised using the gamma detection probe (Fig. 14). The line-of-sight is established as soon as possible and the sentinel node is identified and biopsied as described above.

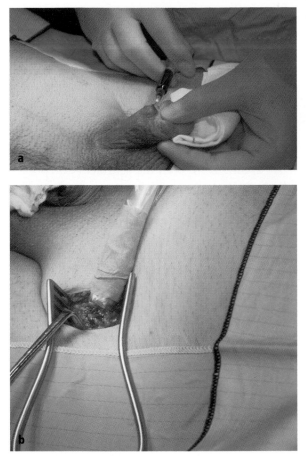

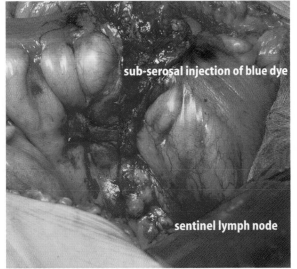

Fig. 15. Sentinel node localisation using blue dye in a patient with sigmoid carcinoma

Fig. 14. **a** Injection of patent blue dye in the dorsum of the penis in a patient who had circumcision as part of treatment of penile carcinoma. **b** Sentinel node biopsy using the Neoprobe 1500

Sentinel Node Biopsy in Colorectal Carcinoma

The relevance of the sentinel node concept in colorectal cancer and the injection technique are described in Chap. 5. In a study performed by Saha and associates on 30 consecutive patients, comprising 25 with colon and 5 with rectal carcinomas [25], sentinel node mapping successfully predicted the lymph node status of the lymphatic basin in 28/30 cases (93.3%). At present this procedure is performed in our institution by intraoperative injection of patent blue dye around the tumour. The mobilisation of the colon is continued and the first node that takes up the blue dye is labelled with a suture as the sentinel node [25] and processed accordingly for histological analysis (Fig. 15).

It has been our experience that in rectal carcinoma, the blue dye moves progressively through all mesorectal lymph nodes, rendering the task of sentinel biopsy difficult (see Chap. 5, Fig. 11 b). Submucosal injection of radiotracer and probe-guided surgery may overcome this problem in the future.

Training Issues

The success of the sentinel node biopsy is operator dependent, as was clearly demonstrated by Krag and associates [12] in a multicentre validation study performed by 11 surgeons in various practice settings. There was significant variation in the success rate achieved by these surgeons, despite their having performed five practice procedures prior to the commencement of the trial: the success rate ranged between 79% and 98%, with a false-negative rate of 0%–29%. There is a definite learning curve associated with this technique. It is extremely important that proper training of surgeons and other members of the multidisciplinary team is ensured before applying this procedure in clinical practice. It is equally important that the data are carefully collected and analysed on a regular basis for quality assurance. Until the uncertainties surrounding various practical issues are resolved, it is desirable that sentinel node biopsy is performed in a trial setting.

Sterilisation and Decontamination Techniques

Most intra-operative probes have been designed to allow gas sterilisation in ethylene oxide if the manufacturer's recommended protocols are followed, and some specific modular probes may even be autoclaved. However, sterilisation may require the probe to be sent to the hospital's central sterilisation service, leading to a delay before the probe is again ready for use; furthermore, the probe is also exposed to the risk of improper handling whilst in transit. Many users therefore choose to encase both the probe and its cable inside a sterile latex cover designed for intraluminal ultrasound probes [26] or, if this is not available, within a sterile glove enclosed in a continuous length of suitable sterile clear plastic tubing. This is then sealed at the probe end using strong surgical tape to prevent blood or tissue from collecting in the folds of the drape, and must be of sufficient length to cover the entire section of cable that may be brought into contact with the assembly of drapes defining the sterile field. Sterile draping of the probe is easy to organise, requiring no prior preparation, and allows for multiple procedures within a single theatre session.

Control units are not designed to be made sterile, and should be placed on a suitable non-sterile trolley sited away from the sterile field and where the visual indicators may be clearly seen by the surgeon performing the procedure. It is advisable to tether the sterile portion of the detector cable to the sterile drapes, thus preventing the probe from an accidental fall whilst in use.

If it is used sterile and uncovered, the probe may become slightly contaminated by the tracer. Initial wiping with a cloth moistened with 70% isopropyl alcohol, followed by a further wipe using a damp cloth soaked in a suitable radioactive decontaminant solution such as Decon90 or Radiacwash, will remove any surface contamination. The presence of a raised background radiation count may signify some residual contamination; however, more likely alternative causes should first be excluded. The probe should then be thoroughly cleaned using a suitable enzymatic detergent, in accordance with the manufacturer's instructions.

Radiation Safety in the Operating Theatre

Radiation safety issues are discussed in detail in Chap. 8. As far as the theatre environment is concerned, it is important that all surgical and theatre staff are familiar with the local radiation safety guidelines. With respect to the disposal of the radiation waste generated at the time of operation, it is our recommendation that all of the clinical waste arising from both the sentinel node procedure and the primary tumour excision should be safely stored for a period of not less than 3 days before its disposal as non-active waste.

Key Points for Clinical Practice

- Surgical techniques used in the intra-operative detection of the sentinel node vary significantly.
- Probe-guided surgery and blue dye localisation are complementary techniques, and their combined use improves the detection rate.
- In malignant melanoma a combination of dynamic lymphoscintigraphy, intra-operative probe guidance and use of blue dye is associated with a high success rate.
- It is important to ensure that the probe is in good working condition before the operation.
- The probe enables the surgeon to determine the site of the incision by finding the area of maximum focal activity.
- It is good practice to try and establish the "line-of-sight" as soon as a surgical incision is made and to continue the dissection directly in that line.
- Background activity needs to be recorded by aiming the probe away from the injection site.
- One of the greatest advantages of probe-guided surgery is that complete excision of the sentinel node can be verified.
- The probe needs to be applied in all directions with careful recording of the residual activity.
- There is a definite learning period associated with the technique and its success is operator dependent.
- The learning period is shorter if the blue dye and probe techniques are combined.
- Radiation risks to staff and patients are minimal.

- Medical and nursing staff should become familiar with the safe use of ionising radiation.
- Training and a multidisciplinary team approach are the keys to the success of the technique.

References

1. Nopajaroonsri C, Luk SC, Simon GT. Ultrastructure of the normal lymph node. *Am J Pathol* 1971; 65:1–24
2. Tortora GJ, Grabowski SR. *Principles of anatomy and physiology*. New York: Harper-Collins; 1996: 676–678
3. Giuliano AE, Kirgan DM, Guenther JM, Morton DL. Lymphatic mapping and sentinel lymphadenectomy for breast cancer. *Ann Surg* 1994; 220:391–398
4. Krag DN, Weaver DL, Alex JC, Fairbank JT. Surgical resection and radiolocalization of the sentinel lymph node in breast cancer using a gamma probe. *Surg Oncol* 1993; 2:335–340
5. Alex JC, Krag DN. Gamma-probe guided localization of lymph nodes. *Surg Oncol* 1993; 2:137–143
6. Alex JC, Weaver DL, Fairbank JT, Krag DN. Gamma-probe guided lymph node localization in malignant melanoma. *Surg Oncol* 1993; 2:303–308
7. Albertini JJ, Lyman GH, Cox C, Yeatman T, Balducci L, Ku N, Shivers S, Berman C, Wells K, Rapaport D, Shons A, Horton J, Greenberg H, Nicosia S, Clark R, Cantor A, Reintgen DS. Lymphatic mapping and sentinel node biopsy in the patient with breast cancer. *JAMA* 1996; 276:1818–1822
8. Veronesi U, Paganelli G, Galimberti V, Viale G, Zurrida ST, Bodeni N, Costa A, Chicco C, Geraghty JG, Luine A, Sacchini V, Veronesi P. Sentinel-node biopsy to avoid axillary dissection in breast cancer with clinically negative lymph-nodes. *Lancet* 1997; 349:1864–1867
9. Giuliano AE, Kirgan DM, Guenther JM, Morton DL. Lymphatic mapping and sentinel lymphadenectomy for breast cancer. *Ann Surg* 1994; 220:391–398
10. Giuliano AE, Jones RC, Brennan M, Statman R. Sentinel lymphadenectomy in breast cancer. *J Clin Oncol* 1997; 15:2345–2350
11. Pijpers R, Meijer S, Hoekstra OS, Collet GJ, Comans FI, Boom RP, van Diest PJ, Teule GJ. Impact of lymphoscintigraphy on sentinel node identification with technetium-99m-colloidal albumin in breast cancer. *J Nucl Med* 1997; 38:366–368
12. Krag D, Weaver D, Ashikaga T, Moffat F, Klimberg VS, Shriver C, Feldman S, Kusminsky R, Gadd M, Kuhn J, Harlow S, Beitsch P. The sentinel node in breast cancer, a multicenter validation study. *N Engl J Med* 1998; 339:941–946
13. Gulec SA, Moffat FL, Carroll RG, Serafini AN, Sfakianakis GN, Allen L, Boggs J, Escobedo D, Pruett CS, Gupta A, Livingstone AS, Krag DN. Sentinel lymph node localization in early breast cancer. *J Nucl Med* 1998; 39:1388–1393
14. Krag D, Harlow S, Weaver D, Ashikaga T. Technique of sentinel node resection in melanoma and breast cancer: probe guided surgery and lymphatic mapping. *Eur J Surg Oncol* 1998; 24:89–93
15. Rodier JF, Janser JC. Surgical technical details improving sentinel node identification in breast cancer. *Oncol Rep* 1997; 4:281–283
16. Borgstein PJ, Pijpers R, Comans EF, van Diest PJ, Boom RP, Meijer S. Sentinel lymph node biopsy in breast cancer: guidelines and pitfalls of lymphoscintigraphy and gamma probe detection. *J Am Coll Surg* 1998; 186:275–283
17. Krag DN, Ashikaga T, Harlow SP, Weaver DL. Development of sentinel node targeting technique in breast cancer patients. *Breast* 1998; 4:67–74
18. Morton DL, Wen D, Wong JH et al. Technical details of intraoperative lymphatic mapping for early stage melanoma. *Arch Surg* 1992; 127:392–399
19. Noguchi M, Kawahara F, Tsugawa K et al. Sentinel lymphadenectomy in breast cancer: an alternative to routine axillary dissection. *Breast Cancer* 1998; 5:1–6
20. O'Hea BJ, Hill AD, El-Shirbiny AM, Yeh SD, Rosen PP, Coit DG, Borgen PI, Cody HS. Sentinel lymph node biopsy in breast cancer: initial experience at Memorial Sloan-Kettering Cancer Center. *J Am Coll Surg* 1998; 186:423–427
21. Uren RF, Howman-Giles RB, Thompson JF. The value of pre-operative lymphoscintigraphy in breast cancer treatment. *Eur J Cancer* 1998; 34:203–204
22. Kapteijn BAE, Nieweg OE, Liem I et al. Localizing the sentinel node in cutaneous melanoma: gamma probe detection versus blue dye. *Ann Surg Oncol* 1997; 4:156–160
23. Cabanas RM. An approach for the treatment of penile carcinoma. *Cancer* 1977; 39:456–466
24. Pijpers R, Borgstein PJ, Meijer S et al. Sentinel node biopsy in melanoma patients: dynamic lymphoscintigraphy followed by intraoperative gamma probe and vital dye guidance. *World J Surg* 1997; 21:788–793
25. Saha S, Espinosa M, Gauthier J, Morrison A, Rohatgi C, Dorman S, Ganatra BK, Desai D, Arora M. Diagnostic and therapeutic implications of sentinel node mapping in colorectal cancer. 51st Society of Surgical Oncology, 1st World Federation of Surgical Oncology Societies Cancer Symposium, San Diego, Calif, March 26–29, 1998: p 31
26. Perkins A. Peroperative nuclear medicine. *Eur J Nucl Med* 1993; 20:573–575
27. McMasters KM, Giuliano AE, Ross MI et al. Sentinel-lymph-node biopsy for breast cancer – not yet the standard of care. *N Engl J Med* 1998; 339:990–995

CHAPTER 8

Dosimetry and Radiation Protection

Introduction

In respect of radiation safety the sentinel node technique has a great advantage in that it requires the injection of relatively low levels of tracer activity. As such the technique conveys little radiation risk to the patient receiving the investigation or to any of the staff groups involved in performing the procedure, whether in the nuclear medicine department, the operating theatre or the histopathology laboratory. Establishing the sentinel node procedure as a routinely performed diagnostic technique should entail only a minimal revision of existing arrangements for radiation protection. However, radiation must always be used in the safest manner possible, and to ensure this the operator needs to adhere both to common sense radiation protection principles and to the relevant legislative requirements.

This chapter is intended as an introduction to the topics of radiation dosimetry and radiation safety as applied to the sentinel node technique, and the prospective user is strongly advised to consult with both the hospital nuclear medicine department and the locally appointed radiation protection adviser (RPA) for further specific advice and information, particularly regarding local radiation protection arrangements.

Principles of Radiation Dosimetry

The SI unit of absorbed radiation dose is the Gray (Gy), defined as the deposition of 1 Joule of energy per kilogram absorbing medium (e.g. body tissue). The Gray replaces the rad, although the latter unit is still often used. This quantity does not take account of the relative biological damage to tissue that is caused by the specific type of radiation effecting the dose, and for this reason a unit termed the equivalent dose is also defined, calculated by multiplying the absorbed radiation dose by a radiation weighting factor w_R as defined by the International Commission on Radiological Protection (ICRP 60 [1]). The SI unit for this quantity is the Sievert (Sv), where this replaces the rem. The radiation weighting factors are listed in Table 1, and it can be seen that the factor for X-rays, gamma rays and beta particles is 1, giving an equivalent dose for these radiations numerically equal to the absorbed dose.

When a radiopharmaceutical is administered to a human subject the internal radiation dose to the body may be estimated by observing its subsequent behaviour. The resulting dose can be shown to depend upon a large number of variables. These range from the physical properties of the radionuclide itself and the radioactivity of the tracer and the route of its administration, to the subject's weight, gender and age, and the biodistribution of the labelled tracer (including the kinetics of tracer uptake and its clearance from each targeted organ or system). The existence of any free or unlabelled radionuclide or the presence of any physiologically active agent or disease state can also effect an influence upon the body's handling of the

Table 1. Radiation weighting factors for different types of radiation

Type of radiation	Radiation weighting factor (w_T)
X-rays, γ-rays, electrons	1
Protons	5
Thermal neutrons	5
Fast neutrons	5–20 (dependent on energy)
α-Particles, fission fragments	20

Table 2. Tissue weighting factors used in the dosimetric concepts of effective dose equivalent and effective dose

Specified organ or tissue	Tissue weighting factor (w_T) for effective dose	Tissue weighting factor (w_T) for effective dose equivalent
Gonads	0.20	0.25
Lung	0.12	0.12
Red bone marrow	0.12	0.12
Stomach	0.12	Not specified
Colon	0.12	Not specified
Thyroid	0.05	0.03
Liver	0.05	Not specified
Oesophagus	0.05	Not specified
Breast	0.05	0.15
Bladder	0.05	Not specified
Skin	0.01	Not specified
Bone surfaces	0.01	0.03
Remaining organs	0.05	0.30
Total	1.00	1.00

tracer, e.g. in the patient with renal failure or the subject administered a thyroid "blocking" agent.

The level of radiation risk arising from differing forms of exposure has been assessed by the International Commission on Radiological Protection (ICRP). In 1977 they introduced the concept of the effective dose equivalent (EDE) (ICRP 26) [2]. This is defined as the sum of the calculated equivalent doses for a set of specified body organs, where each contributing organ dose is multiplied by a tissue weighting factor w_T to account for the relative radiosensitivity for that organ, thereby arriving at a total "effective" whole-body radiation absorbed dose. Subsequently the effective dose (ICRP 60 [1]) has been defined by the ICRP to supersede use of the effective dose equivalent in respect of medical exposures. Although it has a similar underlying concept it incorporates both revised tissue weighting factors and a modified set of specified organs better reflecting the whole patient population. The effective dose has not been completely accepted as a replacement for the effective dose equivalent, however, and in practice both quantities are still in use for dosimetric purposes. By using either, the radiation dose resulting from different radiopharmaceutical administrations may be compared, both with each other and also with the dose resulting from an equivalent exposure caused by uniform irradiation of the whole body. The organs specified in the definitions for both effective dose equivalent and effective dose and their respective tissue weighting factors are shown in Table 2.

However, neither quantity is universally endorsed for dosimetric use by the nuclear medicine community [3], and some authorities still advocate use of the equivalent radiation dose to individual organs only.

A system for calculating the absorbed radiation dose resulting from a radiopharmaceutical administration has been devised by the Medical Internal Radiation Dose (MIRD) Committee of the Society of Nuclear Medicine [4], and is the most widely used and accepted methodology for estimating the radiation dose to human subjects. This schema specifies a set of anthropomorphic human models, both male and female, adult and paediatric. Computer simulations have been run for many distributions of radioactivity within the body organs of these phantoms, yielding data on the relative irradiation between and within the individual source organs. Thus individual organ radiation doses may be determined for any specific administered radionuclide and observed pattern of biodistribution and clearance. From these individual organ doses the effective dose equivalent and effective dose may then be determined.

Sentinel Lymph Node Dosimetry

Radiation dosimetry for the technique of lymphoscintigraphy has been determined by Bergqvist et al. [5]. Their findings indicate an effective dose equivalent of 5.32×10^{-3} mSv/MBq for a subcutaneous injection of ^{99m}Tc-antimony sulphur colloid. An effective dose equivalent of 1.25×10^{-2} mSv/MBq [6] for general diagnostic lymphoscintigraphy procedures is used for licensing purposes in the United Kingdom. However, the route of tracer administration for the sentinel node mapping technique differs significantly from that used for conventional lymphoscintigraphy, where a direct injection of tracer into the lymphatic system is performed, usually into a distal site in the limbs. In the sentinel node mapping procedure the tracer is injected either subdermally, peritumorally or, by some workers, intratumorally (see Chap. 5), and so the tracer here will drain from the site of administration to a much more limited extent. Dosimetry for this technique is therefore expected to differ from that for conventional lymphoscintigraphy for this and a number of other reasons. Radiation dosimetry specific to the sentinel node technique merits further consideration, and the dose received from the application of this procedure to breast cancer is estimated here from patients investigated at our institution.

From our own mammary sentinel node data, where a subdermal injection technique is adopted we have seen a complete absence of any migration of the tracer (Albures) through the lymphatic system beyond the sentinel node, or when visualised, the second-echelon axillary lymph nodes. Our measurements of the activity retained within excised sentinel nodes demonstrate decay-corrected tracer retention in the range 0.005 % – 5 % injected dose at 24 h post-injection. Critical examination of the scintigraphic images obtained have shown no evidence of the specific uptake of tracer into either the bloodstream or the reticuloendothelial system; there is an absence of any vascular activity and no tracer uptake is observed in the liver, spleen or bone marrow of any patient. Blood samples have been taken at varying timepoints between 1 and 48 h post-injection in a number of patients. The samples obtained (2 ml whole blood) were assayed in a gamma well counter calibrated to allow a direct determination of the ^{99m}Tc activity. Very low activity levels were recorded for all of the blood samples taken, indicating an activity concentration lower than 1% of the injected dose within the total circulating blood volume.

For dosimetric purposes, therefore, we have considered that a negligible quantity of tracer leaves the injection site(s), and consequently all tracer is considered to be retained as a localised activity source remaining within the tissue of the breast itself. Pivotal to the sentinel node biopsy technique, the sentinel node itself will always be excised at operation. Breast tissue which retains most of the administered activity may be completely excised (as when a mastectomy is performed), or may be left in situ if a less radical surgical procedure is adopted. The exact extent of the radiation burden to the patient is therefore dependent upon the specific surgical procedure followed, and for the purposes of dosimetry it is assumed here that all tissue retaining the active tracer is left in situ. Removal of this tissue at operation will of course act to reduce the already low radiation dose to the patient.

We have used the data obtained to model the radiation dosimetry for a mammary sentinel node investigation and, more specifically, for the administration of a small volume of ^{99m}Tc-labelled colloid into the subdermal layer of the breast immediately overlying the primary breast tumour. The relative radiosensitivity of breast tissue is also considered in a determination of the effective dose equivalent and effective dose.

Summarising the above findings, some key assumptions have been made:

1. 100 % activity is administered directly into the tissue of the breast.
2. There is negligible biological clearance of radio-activity, either colloidally bound or as free ^{99m}Tc pertechnetate.

Established MIRD methodology has been used to provide a basis for the estimation of individual organ doses, whole-body absorbed radiation dose and the effective dose equivalent and effective dose. All dosimetric indices were determined for the adult non-pregnant female reference model; total body weight 58 kg, with breast tissue totalling 407 g including overlying skin. The MIRDOSE 3.1 software package (Oak Ridge Institute for Science and Education, Oak Ridge, TN 37831), detailed by Stabin [7] was used to perform some of the dose calculations.

Radiation dose to the breast is considered here in terms of both the estimated mean dose to the total breast tissue and the estimated maximum local dose received solely by that tissue absorbing the retained tracer (i.e. that tissue comprising the administration volume after some modest dissemination). Since the average range of ^{99m}Tc gamma rays in soft tissue is approximately 50 mm, it can reasonably be considered that all breast tissue other than that containing the tracer will receive a reasonably uniform radiation dose. On this basis, the classical MIRD dosimetry model has been used to estimate the radiation dose to the total breast.

This standard MIRD model assumes that the tracer is homogeneously distributed throughout the entire tissue of both breasts. This may be refined so as to be more appropriate to the dose estimate for a sentinel node administration by multiplying the calculated dose by a factor of 2 to take account of tracer administration into the affected breast only. This relatively simplistic dose-scaling approach may be considered valid if the relative magnitude of the MIRD-derived geometrical weighting factors ("S-factors") for radiation dose due to cross-irradiation and self-irradiation are considered ("cross-irradiation" is defined as irradiation of the tissue of the contralateral breast due to tracer activity within the breast containing the administered dose, and "self-irradiation" refers to the dose received by the tissue of the affected breast owing to local irradiation from the administered tracer volume itself). The relevant dose weighting factor for "self-dose" will be at least an order of magnitude higher than the dose across to the contralateral breast; thus the latter component to breast dose can be safely ignored. As a further check the radiation dose due to self-irradiation by a homogeneous distribution of activity within an idealised 200-g spherical organ differs from the scaled dose by less than 5%.

Applying this modification then, the resulting mean radiation dose to the tissue of the affected breast is 7.20×10^{-1} mGy/MBq, equating to a dose of 10.8 mGy (0.0108 Gy) for an administered activity of 15 MBq, as performed for our routine sentinel node mapping protocol. Breast tissue totalling in excess of the somewhat low figure of 204 g per breast represented by the MIRD model will receive a lower mean radiation dose; tissue comprising a smaller breast will correspondingly receive a larger mean dose.

Radiation doses for other body organs may also be determined using standard MIRD methodology. The largest of these are to the lung, which receives a dose of 7.79×10^{-3} mGy/MBq, and to the thymus gland, which receives a dose of 9.87×10^{-3} mGy/MBq. These doses result in a total lung dose of 0.12 mGy and a total dose to the thymus gland of 0.15 mGy for an administered activity of 15 MBq. Additionally, if the left breast is investigated then the myocardium will receive a radiation dose approximating to 2×10^{-2} mGy/MBq, or 0.32 mGy per administered dose (if the right breast is investigated then the increased distance between the tissue of the right breast and the myocardium will act to reduce the resulting myocardial radiation dose by a factor of approximately 10 by comparison with a tracer injection into the left breast).

In considering the mean radiation dose to both breasts, the effective dose equivalent is estimated as 5.7×10^{-2} mSv/MBq, and the effective dose as 2.11×10^{-2} mSv/MBq, resulting in an effective dose equivalent of 0.86 mSv and an effective dose of 0.32 mSv for a 15 MBq administration. These values differ largely due to the variation in the tissue weighting factor accorded to breast tissue in the definitions of each quantity (Table 2).

Standard MIRD methodology does, however, assume in this instance that the tracer activity is homogeneously distributed throughout the tissue of the breast. As discussed, this is not true for the sentinel node technique, where the injection technique for 0.1 ml total volume of tracer results in a subdermal or peritumoural bolus deposition after the tracer solution has been injected and disseminated locally by the recommended massaging procedure. The radiation dose received by the small volume of breast tissue retaining the tracer solution will therefore be somewhat higher than that received by the remaining breast tissue. This specified retention volume has been determined at our institution for a sample of 12 patients receiving a subdermal administration for sentinel node investigation of carcinoma of the breast. Measurements of tracer distribution obtained from images acquired at 1 h post-injection indicate with good intersubject agreement that the volume appears to be 2–5 ml, dependent upon whether tracer dispersion is considered to be constrained to a thin (4 mm) subdermal layer or to occur throughout a more arbitrary deeper hemispherical volume. The resulting dose will be approximately 20- to 50-fold higher than the estimated radiation dose to the whole breast, i.e. 14–36 mGy/MBq.

These data are in good agreement with those of Bergqvist [5], who determined radiation doses arising from the subcutaneous injection of ^{99m}Tc-antimony sulphur colloid for the investigation of malignant melanoma and also with the findings of Bronskill in 1983 [8], who determined the radiation dose to local tissue resulting from an interstitial injection of ^{99m}Tc-antimony sulphur colloid to investigate the internal mammary chain. Bergqvist reported a mean absorbed dose to the injection site of 9.46 mGy/MBq with a maximum dose of about 40 mGy/MBq, and Bronskill calculated a mean absorbed dose of 27.4 mGy/MBq, each finding having been obtained from the application of MIRD methodology to scintigraphic observations of the kinetics of tracer clearance from the injection site.

The localised radiation dose to the breast tissue comprising the administered volume should, however, be considered in this context in relation to its subsequent fate – either that of complete excision at operation or the normal practice of postoperative exposure to a course of external beam radiotherapy, where a radiation dose of 50 Gy to the breast and axilliary lymph node fields is typically prescribed.

With a similar volume and the range of tracer uptakes reported above, the sentinel lymph node itself will receive a maximum dose of approximately 5% of that received by the breast tissue within the tracer administration volume, and it will moreover be excised from the body to enable the sentinel node biopsy to be performed.

Dosimetry for the sentinel node procedure in malignant melanoma will result in a radiation dose dependent upon the exact location of the tumour, and upon the fractionation of the injection, the total volume and eventual dissemination of the administered tracer. However, as the primary tumour is located in the cutaneous layer the radiosensitivity of this tissue is significantly lower than for the breast (Table 2) and accordingly both the effective dose equivalent and the effective dose will be lower than for an administration to the breast. Additionally, the injection site(s) are significantly more likely to be excised at operation.

Table 3. Effective dose for a number of nuclear medicine and radiological investigations (data obtained from the National Radiological Protection Board (NRPB)

Investigation	Effective dose (mSv)
Sentinel node technique (ca. breast)	0.32
Technetium-99m bone scan	3.6
Technetium-99m lung perfusion scan	1.0
Iodine-123 thyroid scan	4.4
Mammography (four films)	0.4
Chest X-ray	0.04
Abdominal X-ray	1.5
Barium meal	5.0
Lumbar spine X-ray	2.4
Intravenous urography	4.6
Abdominal CT	7.2
Chest CT	8.3
Brain CT	1.8

ca., Carcinoma; CT, computed tomography.

Comparative Radiation Doses

Table 3 shows the estimated effective dose for the sentinel node mapping procedure in carcinoma of the breast against that resulting from a number of commonly performed nuclear medicine and radiographic procedures. Table 4 lists the radiation dose resulting from a number of causes, both natural and man-made. The total detriment arising from an effective dose of 1 mSv has been suggested by the ICRP (ICRP 60 [1]) to be 73 per million (where detriment is defined as the total risk due to the induction of all cancers, both fatal and non-fatal, and of severe hereditary effects), and the risk of fatal cancer induction to be 50 per million. This equates to a total detriment for the 0.32 mSv effective dose resulting from the sentinel lymph node procedure of 23.4 per million, or 1 in 42 808, and a risk of fatal cancer of 16 per million or 1 in 62 500. Table 5 lists a number of everyday life activities carrying a risk equal to the risk of fatal cancer induction per mSv.

Principles of Radiation Protection

It is a fundamental principle of radiation protection that radiation exposures must be justified. This applies both to occupational exposures received resulting from work practices involving the

Table 4. Radiation dose arising from the sentinel node technique, compared with a range of natural and man-made sources and statutory dose limits (data obtained from the National Radiological Protection Board (NRPB)

Source of radiation exposure/relevant legislative limits	Radiation dose (mSv)
Sentinel node technique (ca. breast)	0.32
Return airflight: London to New York (dose from cosmic rays)	0.06
Return airflight: London to Sydney (dose from cosmic rays)	0.20
Annual UK dose from natural radioactivity in food and drink	0.37
Two weeks residence in Cornwall, UK (additional dose from radon gas emanating from granite geology)	0.25
One year's residence in Denver, USA (additional radiation dose from cosmic radiation at higher altitude)	0.88
Average total UK annual radiation dose to the public (all causes)	2.6
Proposed annual UK dose limit to the public (ICRP 60, 1990)	1.0
Existing annual UK dose limit to the public (IRR, 1985)	5.0
Proposed annual UK dose limit for a radiation worker (ICRP 60, 1990)	20
Existing annual UK dose limit for a radiation worker (IRR, 1985)	50

Table 5. Life activities having a risk of fatality equal to that due to cancer induction per mSv radiation dose (data from Shields and Lawson [9] and Pochin [10])

Equivalent sources of fatal risk
1 mSv effective radiation dose Smoking 75 cigarettes Drinking 1 glass of wine daily for 6 months Travelling 125 miles by motorcycle Travelling 2500 miles by car Travelling 16000 miles by airplane Rock climbing for 75 min Canoeing for 5 h

use of radiation, and to exposures made for medical reasons. In the case of medical exposures this justification must be both for the individual concerned and for the type of examination itself. Furthermore, all forms of exposure should be "as low as reasonably practicable, social and economic factors taken into account" – this is often termed the "ALARP" principle.

United Kingdom Radiation Protection Legislation and Its Implementation

Within the United Kingdom, use of radiation falls under the requirements of the Ionising Radiations Regulations 1985 [11] of the Health and Safety at Work Act (1974) and its associated documents. It is the responsibility of the individual employing authority to ensure compliance with this legislation; within the public sector this is defined as the Chief Executive of the NHS Trust. The employing authority *appoints* one (or more) Radiation Protection Advisor (RPA), an expert in the field of radiological safety, and *may* administer radiation safety policy through a Radiation Safety Committee. Within each individual department or specialist unit a Radiation Protection Supervisor (RPS) is further appointed to be responsible for the direct management of local radiation safety arrangements, within overall guidelines set by the RPA. These take the form of approved Local Rules for Radiation Safety, which must be followed and are subjected to regular updates. Annual radiation dose limits for both radiation workers and the public are also set by the Regulations, and for this purpose hospital employees not routinely brought into contact with radiation by the nature of their employment are treated as members of the public. In relation to implementation of the sentinel node technique this will include both operating theatre and pathology laboratory staff. These Regulations are currently under review as a result of a revision of the governing EC Basic Safety Standards Directive that brought about their formulation and, at press, are due to be superseded by May 2000.

Medical exposures are further controlled by the Ionising Radiation (Protection of the Patient Undergoing Medical Examination or Treatment) Regulations 1988 (POPUMET) [12]. This defines two key roles in the making of a medical radiation exposure, and requires that both individuals be named for all procedures performed. The first role is that of the "clinical director", a suitably experienced clinician responsible for justification of the exposure, and the second role is filled by a person qualified as competent to actually perform or "physically direct" the exposure – for nuclear medicine procedures the person actually injecting the radioactive tracer is defined as having physically directed the exposure. A suitable single individual may be qualified to perform both roles. Unless already professionally trained, as for example a radiographer, holders of both roles are required to hold a certificate indicating that they have received an appropriate training in radiation protection, popularly known as the "POPUMET certificate"; this may be gained by attendance at a one-day training course. These regulations are currently also under review, and a revised Medical Exposures Directive is expected to be passed as legislation in the UK by May 2000.

The medical administration of radioactive products is subject to the Medicines (Administration of Radioactive Substances) Regulations 1978 [13]. These require the clinician responsible for a radionuclide investigation to hold certificate(s) issued by the Administration of Radioactive Substances Advisory Committee (ARSAC) of the Department of Health, indicating that the holder has sufficient appropriate experience to prescribe radiopharmaceuticals in support of the investigations specified under that certificate. Separate licences are held for diagnostic and therapeutic procedures, and an investigation made for the purposes of research requires a application to the committee for a specific further licence.

Arrangements for the storage and disposal of radioactive products are controlled by the Radioactive Substances Act (1993) [14]. All hospital sites receiving, holding and disposing of radioactive materials require appropriate Registration and Authorisation under this Act. Licences are issued and administered by the UK Environment Agency. Transport of radioactive materials is similarly subject to the Radioactive Material (Road Transport) (Great Britain) Regulations 1996 [15].

Practical Radiation Protection Implementation

Two forms of exposure risk exist when unsealed sources of gamma emitting radiation are present. The first is that of external irradiation, when an

Table 6. Indices relevant to radiation protection for ^{99m}Tc

Half-life of radioactive decay	6.02 h
Energy of gamma ray emission	140 keV
Half value layer (HVL) for soft tissue	46 mm
Half value layer (HVL) for lead shielding	0.17 mm
Tenth value layer (TVL) for lead shielding	0.9 mm

individual's proximity to the radioactive source leads to their radiation exposure by the gamma rays emitted from the source and absorbed by the body tissues of the individual. The second arises from the exposure that results when there is an accidental intake of radioactive material due to direct contact with a source of radiation leading to the ingestion, inhalation or skin absorption of radioactivity.

The risk from external irradiation may be reduced, often dramatically, by consideration of three key factors: time, distance and shielding (the "TDS rule"). For a constant radiation dose rate arising from proximity to a source of radiation the individual may reduce the resulting exposure by minimising contact time with the radiation source, by increasing their distance from the source, or by shielding the source with an absorptive medium. The second factor observes the "inverse square law", in that the radiation dose rate, and therefore the relative risk, falls by a factor equal to the square of the intervening distance. As an example the dose rate at a distance of 1 m is one-hundredth that of the dose rate at 10 cm. Use of a shielding material reduces the dose rate according to the exponential relationship outlined in Chap. 3. Table 6 indicates a number of indices relevant to radiation protection for unsealed sources of ^{99m}Tc.

The internal radiation exposure risk due to the accidental intake of radioactivity by ingestion, inhalation or skin absorption is minimised by the adoption of good radiation protection practice and universal surgical precautions, and should normally present an insignificant hazard to all staff groups involved.

Good Radiation Protection Practice When Injecting the Tracer

The radioactive tracer will normally be injected within the nuclear medicine department, where suitable facilities exist for its administration and for the safe handling and disposal of the radioactive waste produced. Additionally, as radiation workers the departmental staff involved are professionally trained in the principles and practice of radiation protection relating to unsealed sources of radioactivity. Existing mandatory Local Rules for Radiation Safety will cover all relevant arrangements and requirements. The injection technique outlined in Chap. 5 incorporates all the requirements for good radiation protection practice at this pivotal stage of the procedure, and if followed, the risk to both patient and staff of direct contamination by the radioactive tracer should be very low. The increase in occupational radiation exposure to the departmental staff arising from the very low levels of radioactivity used in this investigation should be negligible.

Good Radiation Protection Practice in the Operating Theatre

The patient is usually scheduled for operation between 4 and 24 h after tracer administration. When radioactive decay is taken into account this results in an activity of between 1 and 10 MBq retained at the injection site by the time the operation is performed. As detailed earlier, with the exception of the sentinel node and other axillary lymph nodes demonstrating a similar level of tracer uptake there will be a negligible distribution of radioactivity external to the injection site. Specifically, there is an absence of detectable radioactivity both in the general circulation and in unrelated body tissues.

In considering the possibility for radiation risk, however remote, potentially both internal and external radiation exposure may arise. Staff may be irradiated by virtue of their proximity to the radioactive patient, and may also come into direct contact with the radioactive tracer in vivo, or with any excised radioactive tissue specimen or contaminated dressings, drapes or operating theatre equipment.

The maximum activity retained within the injection site at the time of operation will be approximately 10 MBq ^{99m}Tc. Exposure to an *unattenuated* (i.e. unshielded) radioactive source containing this activity will effect a radiation dose

rate of 0.17×10^{-6} Sv (0.17 μSv) per hour at a distance of 1 m from the source, and 1.8 μSv/h at 30 cm distance (using dose rate data obtained from the Institute of Physical Sciences in Medicine (IPSM, Report No. 63) [16]. For each surgical procedure, a typical total exposure time to the tissue containing the injection site of 1 h, at the lesser distance, will result in a maximum radiation dose to the surgeon(s) involved of approximately 1.8 μSv per patient procedure. The maximum permitted annual radiation dose to a member of the public (this definition is also applicable to any member of staff not formally designated as a radiation worker) will be reduced in the UK in the year 2000 to 1 mSv (ICRP 60) [1], thereby allowing approximately *500 sentinel node procedures to be performed per year* according to the protocol detailed in this text before the individual exposed approaches this annual dose limit. It may be seen, therefore, that a very low external radiation hazard exists to members of staff. One circumstance requiring extra consideration may be that of the pregnant female surgeon or scrub nurse if they perform this procedure regularly as specific lower dose limits apply to the pregnant worker in respect of the radiation dose to the foetus. The issuing of personal radiation badges to staff would be useful in resolving the exact significance of this issue, given individual local circumstances of both workload and surgical protocols.

All theatre staff in contact with either the patient or excised radioactive tissue should be prevented from direct physical contact with the radioactive tracer by the observation of standard bio-hazard precautions, i.e. by wearing protective clothing such as surgical or protective gloves and theatre greens. The intra-operative probe is usually contained within a secure sterile cover and will not therefore become contaminated by any tracer with which it comes into contact. If used when sterilised, a specified decontamination procedure may be performed prior to preliminary disinfection of the probe after use. However, contamination should normally be at a low level. All excised tissue specimens should be bagged or placed in a suitable specimen container for transport to the histopathology laboratory immediately following excision, and the package should be clearly marked as belonging to a patient receiving a ^{99m}Tc sentinel node procedure. There is a negligible risk to personnel involved in this task.

By following these practices, it should be possible to prevent the possibility of an unintentional internal intake of radioactivity. The annual limits of intake (ALI) for a member of the public arising from accidental occupational ingestion and inhalation of ^{99m}Tc are set at 45 MBq and 35 MBq respectively (ICRP 68) [17]. To approach either ALI, activities greater than that contained within the maximum total administration of tracer would need to be accidentally ingested or inhaled by an individual member of staff; an event regarded as extremely unlikely to occur in one single contamination incident, from whatever cause this contamination may arise. Cumulative internal contamination consistent with these annual limits is also regarded as an extremely unlikely event.

Radioactive contamination by bodily fluids, sterile dressings, drapes or theatre equipment is normally negligible owing to the insignificant movement of tracer activity outside the injection site. One notable and very significant exception has, however, been found to this general situation. Should the operative procedure require that the tissue incorporating the administered tracer be surgically dissected then such sterile gauze swabs as are used to absorb blood shed directly from this tissue may also absorb a measurable portion of the administered activity. A number of swabs have been recovered and analysed for radioactive content by direct counting using a gamma camera and a small proportion only have been found to demonstrate absorption in excess of 10 % of the injected activity (when corrected for radioactive decay). At the time of operation these contaminated swabs will therefore have absorbed activity levels reaching 0.1 MBq. This activity will be sufficiently absorbed within the fabric itself to constitute a negligible contamination hazard, although caution should be exercised in their repeated use throughout the procedure. If they are kept physically distant from the direct path of investigation when gamma probing is in progress then they should not in themselves lead to erroneously high probe readings but they do represent a potentially significant and unwanted source of activity within the field of sensitivity of the detector probe. With this radioactive content such contaminated swabs must certainly be considered to constitute radioactive clinical waste.

Radiation protection requirements in respect of the handling and disposal of such radioactive waste are perhaps most appropriately met by complying with the following guidelines as routine practice for all patients investigated. All clinical waste arising from both the sentinel node procedure and the primary tumour excision should be collected, sealed and "double-bagged", i.e. contained within two separate suitable plastic bags. The outer bag should be clearly marked as containing radioactive material, and as belonging to a patient who has undergone a ^{99m}Tc sentinel node procedure. This bag should then be safely stored for a period of not less than 3 days until its contents have undergone sufficient radioactive decay to permit its disposal as non-active waste, when all radioactive markings should be removed. Ideally the bag should be removed to the nuclear medicine department for storage, where appropriate shielding arrangements exist for such waste. However, whilst this is the most acceptable and desirable arrangement it is not mandatory, providing suitable storage facilities exist in a clearly demarcated site located remote from active working areas, e.g. an equipment store room. If it can be clearly shown that such arrangements are strictly adhered to, for all procedures, then compliance with legislative practices and disposal limits can be demonstrated to the appropriate inspecting bodies.

Non-disposable theatre equipment will undergo effective decontamination without further risk during subsequent routine re-sterilisation procedures. The intra-operative probe itself should, however, be tested for contamination using a suitably calibrated contamination monitor and decontaminated if required, if it has been previously sterilised and is used without a separate sterile covering (see Chap. 3).

Good Radiation Protection Practice in the Pathology Laboratory

Histopathology staff also have the potential to experience both internal and external radiation exposure by virtue of their work practices. However, if the standard bio-hazard precautions are observed then there should be no direct physical contact with either the excised radiolabelled tumour or sentinel node specimens when these are presented to the laboratory for preparation and examination.

Initial pre-processing of specimens will bring histopathology staff into close physical proximity with the sample itself. The resulting exposure by external irradiation will be as outlined above for theatre staff, once individual workload and pathology protocols are considered. However, the initial sample preparation is typically very rapidly executed and as such should present little scope for any measurable radiation exposure. Subsequent to this initial stage, preparatory fixing of the specimen in formalin for a period of not less than 48 h will lead to a reduction in the radioactive content of the specimen by a factor of approximately 250. Thus normal histological analysis of multiple tissue samples entails negligible further exposure to radiation. After a total of 1 week's storage, all tissue specimens will have decayed such that they will now contain less than 1 Bq activity, and may safely be disposed of as non-radioactive waste. Local radiation protection advice may be profitably sought to assist in planning a suitable scheme of work for the routine decontamination of sectioning equipment used in the initial preparation of the primary tumour specimen. However, providing standard bio-hazard precautions are followed, both the external and the internal radiation hazard to personnel will be negligible.

As outlined previously, extra consideration should be given to the pregnant female histopathologist or pathology technologist, if they are to perform this procedure regularly. The issue of personal radiation badges to relevant staff members will be useful in resolving the exact significance of this issue in the context of local protocols.

Frozen section analysis of sentinel nodes will entail the rapid processing and sectioning of the identified sentinel lymph node(s). At this time they may contain a maximum of approximately 0.5 MBq tracer. External irradiation is of little consequence here; however, as discussed above, the sectioning equipment used to perform the procedure may require routine decontamination prior to its use for subsequent applications. Again, providing universal precautions are adhered to, both the external and internal radiation hazard should be negligible.

Summary of Recommendations for Good Practice

- Inject the tracer in the nuclear medicine department if at all possible.
- Follow recommended injection techniques closely with respect to radiation protection advice.
- If possible obtain dose rate readings in the operating theatre to verify occupational exposure levels for key staff, for an initial representative number of sentinel node procedures performed according to local protocols.
- Take account of the appropriate legislative occupational radiation dose limits in the light of the currently prevailing sentinel node workload.
- Follow routine sterile precautions in the operating theatre whenever tracer-bearing tissue or clinical waste is handled.
- Exercise caution in the continued use of sterile swabs once these have been directly exposed to the injection site.
- Store clinical waste in a safe manner, suitably labelled and located, and for not less than 3 days prior to disposal.
- Mark all histological specimens as arising from a sentinel node procedure.
- Follow storage and disposal guidelines for the pathology laboratory, decontaminating such equipment after use as is considered necessary.

References

1. International Commission on Radiological Protection. 1990 Recommendations of the ICRP. ICRP Publication 60. New York: Pergamon Press, 1990
2. International Commission on Radiological Protection. Recommendations of the ICRP. ICRP Publication 26. New York: Pergamon Press, 1977
3. Poston JW. Application of the effective dose equivalent to nuclear medicine patients. *J Nucl Med* 1993; 34:714–716
4. Loevinger R, Budinger TF, Watson EE. *MIRD primer for absorbed dose calculations.* New York: Society of Nuclear Medicine, 1991
5. Bergqvist L, Strand S-E, Persson B, Hafström L, Jönsson P-E. Dosimetry in lymphoscintigraphy of Tc-99m antimony sulfide colloid. *J Nucl Med* 1982; 23:698–705
6. Administration of Radioactive Substances Advisory Committee (ARSAC). Notes for guidance on the administration of radioactive substances to persons for the purpose of diagnosis, treatment and research. London: Department of Health, 1993
7. Stabin MG. MIRDOSE: personal computer software for internal dose assessment in nuclear medicine. *J Nucl Med* 1996; 37:538–546

8. Bronskill MJ. Radiation dose estimates for interstitial radio-colloid lymphoscintigraphy. *Semin Nucl Med* 1993; 8:20–25

9. Shields RA, Lawson RS. Effective dose equivalent. *Nucl Med Commun* 1987; 8:851–855

10. Pochin EE. Occupational and other fatality rates. *Community Health* 1974; 6:2–13

11. The Ionising Radiations Regulations 1985. London: HMSO (ISBN 0-11-057333-1)

12. The Ionising Radiation (Protection of the Patient Undergoing Medical Examination or Treatment) Regulations 1988. London: HMSO (ISBN 0-11-086778-5)

13. The Medicines (Administration of Radioactive Substances) Regulations 1978. London: HMSO (ISBN 0-11-084006-2)

14. Radioactive Substances Act 1993. London: HMSO (ISBN 0-10-541293-7)

15. The Radioactive Material (Road Transport) (Great Britain) Regulations 1996. London: HMSO (ISBN 0-11-054742-X)

16. Institute of Physical Sciences in Medicine. Goldstone KE, Jackson PC, Myers MJ, Simpson AE, eds. Report No. 63: Radiation protection in nuclear medicine and pathology. York: IPSM, 1991 (ISBN 0-904181-62-6)

17. International Commission on Radiological Protection. Dose coefficients for intakes of radionuclides by workers. ICRP Publication 68. New York: Pergamon Press, 1995

CHAPTER 9

Histopathology of the Sentinel Node

Background

Breast carcinoma is the commonest malignancy in women and it is estimated that 1 in 12 women will develop such a tumour within their lifetime. The multistep model of breast carcinogenesis suggests that tumours arise via clonal expansion with the acquisition of multiple genetic hits that eventually results in an ability to invade stroma and subsequently to produce metastatic disease [1]. As part of this evolution, it has generally been assumed that tumours first metastasise to regional lymph nodes and subsequently to systemic sites. However, the alternative view, that breast cancer is a systemic disease at the outset, has also been proposed [2]; according to this model, breast cancer cells are already present in the systemic circulation before clinically evident lymph node metastases. Although the concept of tumours first metastasising to lymph nodes may be an oversimplification, lymph node status still remains the most important prognostic indicator [3, 4]. Other important prognostic indicators include tumour type, size and grade [5, 6].

The aforementioned four prognostic features are routinely assessed during the histopathological examination of a breast specimen. There are two principal reasons why the data derived from such an examination may be inaccurate:

1. Inter-observer variability in the assessment of the histopathological parameters
2. Inadequacy in the techniques used for the examination

The lay public, as well as many doctors, has difficulty in understanding how examination under the microscope may not reveal an accurate diagnosis. The histopathological examination of tissues is a subjective assessment and prone to inconsis-

tency due to the personal opinion of the histopathologist as well as difficulties in defining features accurately. For instance, the grading system in the breast is assessed by analysing three different features [7]: the proportion of the tumour-forming tubules ($<10\%$, $10\% - 75\%$, $>75\%$), the pleomorphism (difference in size and shape of the nuclei) and mitotic count over ten high power fields (hpf). The hpf will clearly be dependent on the field diameter of the $\times 40$ lens used to assess the slide. To overcome this problem, charts have been created to standardise the cut-off values for the mitotic count for a given field diameter. Although there is an attempt to be objective in such a grading system, it must be quite clear that the assessment of the proportion of tumour showing good tubule formation and the assessment of pleomorphism are still subjective exercises. Variations in mitotic count may also arise depending on which part of the tumour is examined. Consequently, although pathologists agree broadly on the type and grade of tumours, the agreement is by no means perfect. A number of studies have shown that κ-statistics for inter-observer variation for the assessment of tumour type, tumour grade and tumour size are lower than might be predicted without an understanding of the limitations of examination [8, 9].

Variations in the histopathological assessment may also result from the techniques used for the examination of the specimen. Breast cancer is a heterogeneous disease both clinically and morphologically. It is not surprising, therefore, that factors such as the number of sections examined per case could influence the typing and the grading of the tumour. By examining a limited amount of tissue, the proportion of tumour showing good tubule formation, the degree of pleomorphism and the mitotic count could all be underestimated. This is occasionally seen when high-grade invasive ductal carcinoma is present side by side with a lower grade invasive lobular carcinoma. The problem has been further highlighted by the use of Tru-cut biopsies for diagnosis. Occasionally, examination of the resected specimen reveals a marked difference in grade compared with that predicted from the initial small biopsy. These limitations, which are limitations of the techniques used in the examination of tissues, are the principal sources of error in the assessment of lymph node metastasis. Although the lymph node status is the most important prognostic indicator, in most laboratories the assessment of lymph nodes is confined to examination of a single haematoxylin and eosin (H & E) stained section from each node. Is this type of lymph node examination adequate and what are the consequences for the patient?

Lymph Node Examination: Paraffin Sections

It was as long ago as 1948 that Saphir and Amromin [10] demonstrated that serial sectioning of lymph nodes improves the detection of lymph node metastases. In their study, 33% of patients who were initially diagnosed on routine histology as being lymph node-negative were converted to lymph node-positive by the examination of multiple serial sections. This was subsequently confirmed in 1961 by Pickren [11], who demonstrated occult metastases in 22% of node-negative cases. Unfortunately no prognostic significance was demonstrated between the two groups. Between 1971 and 1996, a further 29 studies of micrometastasis have been reported in literature [12–40]. The number of cases has ranged from 5 to 921 (Ludwig Breast Cancer Study Group) and the type of examination has ranged from one haematoxylin and eosin (H & E) section to serial sections of the entire lymph node, with the use of immunohistochemistry for cytokeratins in some cases. The detection rate for occult metastasis has ranged from 7% to 31%. The follow-up period for many studies has been only 2–3 years; however, in one study, it was greater than 16 years [38]. It was not until 1987 that Trojani et al. [23] demonstrated a statistically significant difference in disease-free survival and overall survival in patients with such occult metastases. The next study to confirm such an effect was that

from the Ludwig Breast Cancer Study Group [29], who showed detection of micrometastases in 9% of their patients. Follow-up to 5 years showed a significant difference in the disease-free survival and the overall survival of these patients. The authors concluded that the pathological examination of a single H & E section is "probably no longer clinically tenable". Since then a large number of studies have demonstrated that the detection of occult metastasis within the lymph node has prognostic significance for the patient, and it is quite clear that there is a survival disadvantage for such patients. So what are the implications for the routine examination of lymph nodes from breast cancer specimens?

As mentioned above, it was been known for more than 30 years that the examination of a single section of a lymph node is inadequate for the assessment of lymph node metastasis. Since the lymph node status is an important prognostic indicator, should we now abandon this technique in favour of more extensive lymph node analysis? The immediate problem that arises is how extensive should this investigation be? In the studies reported to date, there has been wide variability in the level of sectioning of the lymph node, ranging from a few levels through the node to complete examination of the node using serial sectioning. The majority of the pathology laboratories within the United Kingdom and around the world would come to a standstill if every single breast cancer case were examined by cutting hundreds of serial sections of every single lymph node that was removed from the patient. Since extensive serial sectioning is clearly not possible for most laboratories, what constitutes a reasonable number of sections for the detection of most occult metastases? Despite the vast number of studies reported in the literature over the past two decades, the answer to this question remains unclear, and the majority of laboratories continue to use a single H & E section to examine lymph nodes.

Use of Immunohistochemistry for the Detection of Micrometastases

There have been at least 17 studies in the past 20 years reporting the use of immunohistochemistry in the diagnosis of occult metastases within

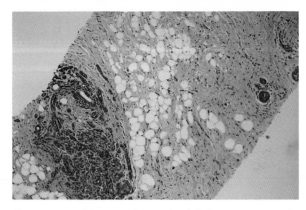

Fig. 1. Tru-cut biopsy with invasive lobular carcinoma. The tumour cells are difficult to see on H & E section

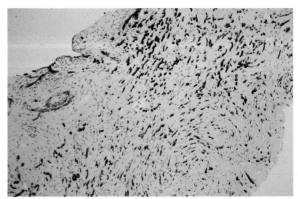

Fig. 2. The invasive lobular carcinoma is highlighted with a cytokeratin marker (MNF 116). The extent of the tumour is much more apparent here than with H & E staining

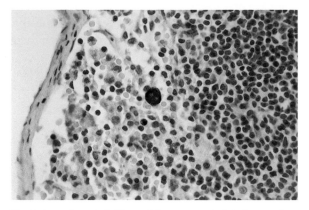

Fig. 3. Lymph node infiltrated by metastatic lobular carcinoma. Single cells may be highlighted by use of cytokeratin stain (MNF 116)

lymph nodes [20–23, 25, 27, 28, 30–32, 34–37, 39, 40]. Monoclonal antibodies for the detection of cytokeratins have been used either alone or in combination with H & E slides in these studies. It is clear that the additional immunohistochemistry improves the detection of micrometastases compared with H & E staining on its own. Not surprisingly perhaps, the technique is particularly useful for certain types of breast carcinoma. Invasive lobular carcinoma is a good example as it tends to infiltrate as either single cells or a small group of cells (Figs. 1–3). Tumour cells from invasive lobular carcinoma are very difficult to differentiate from histiocytes, found as a normal reaction within lymph nodes. Although there is no doubt that immunohistochemistry is superior to H & E sectioning for the detection of such small

occult metastases, it is difficult to envisage the use of immunohistochemistry in the examination of all nodes from the axilla. It is unlikely that such a practice would be implemented in most laboratories. The increase in workload that would occur would not be acceptable to most immunohistochemistry laboratories.

Molecular Techniques for Diagnosis of Lymph Node Metastases

Over the past 5 years, advances in molecular biology have been translated into diagnostic tests for the detection of altered genes or gene products in tumour samples. The advancement in polymerase chain reaction (PCR) – based technology has meant that analysis can also be carried out on paraffin-embedded tissues. It has been demonstrated that reverse transcriptase polymerase chain reaction (RT-PCR) is a sensitive method for the detection of specific gene products in cancer cells [41–46]. The method is extremely sensitive and capable of detecting one cancer cell within a population of 10^6 normal lymph node cells. A number of different gene products, including cytokeratin 19 and Muc 1, have been used for diagnostic purposes. The initial results from such molecular studies look promising and it is clear that molecular techniques are more sensitive in detecting occult lymph node metastases than H & E sectioning either alone or in combination with immunohistochemistry. Currently the main problems with these molecular techniques relate to the occurrence of false-positive and false-negative cases and validation of the techniques as predictors of disease recurrence. False-negative data are likely to occur because of inadequate tissue samples or as a result of technical problems in extracting RNA from paraffin material. Amplification techniques such as those used in RT-PCR are prone to contamination. This has to be controlled for very carefully as false-positive results would clearly mean wrong management for the patient if such data were used in clinical practice. A further compounding problem is that some studies have demonstrated that so-called specific tumour antigens, such as cytokeratin 19 and Muc 1, are also expressed in the blood and lymph nodes of patients without cancer [47]. If these tumour antigens were indeed expressed by normal tissues, then the usefulness of these techniques would be limited. Hence, at present, the value of these techniques in routine diagnostic practice is unclear and awaits clarification.

Sentinel Node Biopsy in Breast Cancer Management

The increasing use of mammographic screening has led to earlier detection of breast cancer, and the detection of small invasive carcinomas and lesions at an earlier stage in development, i.e. ductal carcinoma in situ. Many of these small invasive carcinomas are associated with a negative lymph node status within the axilla. Over the past 20–30 years it has been demonstrated that up to a third of these patients will harbour occult lymph node metastases and that these can be detected by means of serial sectioning, immunohistochemistry and molecular biology techniques using RT-PCR. These small micrometastases have prognostic significance; patients who harbour such metastases have a poorer disease-free survival and overall survival compared with truly lymph node-negative patients.

Since it is clear that the detection of occult metastases has clinical implications, a protocol has to be developed for the incorporation of techniques for their detection within routine diagnostic practice. As stated above, in most laboratories the serial sectioning of every single lymph node and the use of immunohistochemistry on every node are not feasible. Although molecular biology tech-

niques are becoming more widespread, they are unlikely to be used in most district general hospitals and most non-academic units other than for research proposes. Hence it is clear that an alternative strategy will have to be developed for the identification of patients who harbour these occult lymph node metastases. The development of protocols for the identification and sampling of the sentinel node is therefore an advance on past procedures. Since the sentinel node is defined as the first lymph node that drains the primary tumour in the region of the lymphatic basin, it seems logical that examination of this lymph node will be predictive for the rest of the axilla. Is there any evidence that this is indeed the case?

There are now at least 11 studies in the literature that have investigated the role of assessment of the sentinel node in predicting disease within the axilla [48–61]. The number of patients studied ranges from 25 to more than 400. All of these studies claim a specificity and a positive predictive value of 100% and a sensitivity in the range of 88%–100%. The most important feature, however, must be the false-negative rate, i.e. the percentage of patients in whom the sentinel node is negative but the axilla positive. The figures from the studies indicate a false-negative rate ranging from 0% to 12.5%. Questions remain as to what constitutes an acceptable false-negative rate, and further studies will be needed to examine whether special techniques such as immunohistochemistry and molecular techniques can reduce the rate to an "acceptable" level. At University College London (UCL), we are also investigating the role of sentinel node biopsy by use of frozen and paraffin H & E sections and immunohistochemistry.

Protocol for the Examination of Sentinel Nodes at UCL

If the examination of sentinel nodes is to be useful in the management of patients with breast cancer then these nodes will have to be assessed accurately. The studies to date have examined the sentinel node either with the use of a single paraffin section or H & E staining combined with immunohistochemistry. Intra-operative frozen section diagnosis has also been used in some studies but needs further evaluation[48, 62]. If the sentinel node is to be part of the routine surgical management of the patient, it is possible that the surgeon will require a frozen section examination so that the decision regarding resection of the axilla can be made at the time of the primary operation. Routine paraffin section examination with or without immuno-histochemistry might mean that some patients would require a further anaesthetic procedure to deal with the axilla.

Our research protocol involves the use of frozen section followed by confirmatory paraffin section. Pathology examination of the axillary dissection is at present dealt with routinely. If the sentinel node is negative on both frozen section and paraffin section, a pan-cytokeratin marker (MNF 116) is used to check for micrometastases. The data from the sentinel node are then correlated with the axillary dissection.

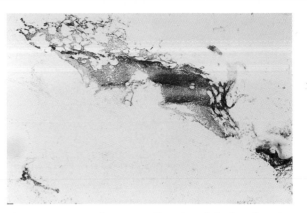

Fig. 4. Extensive replacement of lymph node by fat. Obtaining good quality frozen sections with clear architecture and cytological detail is difficult

Frozen Section

At our institution, the sentinel node is identified and placed separately in a container and brought fresh to the pathology laboratory. The lymph node is examined within 30 min of removal and is kept on ice during the transport. The gross measurements and appearance of the node are recorded and it is bisected into two pieces. Both halves are placed onto the chuck containing OCT (optimum cutting temperature) compound and frozen using cryo-spray. The lymph node is then sectioned at three levels (hence a total of six levels) and stained with H & E. All frozen sections are examined by the same histopathologist with an interest in breast disease. The findings are recorded without knowledge of the axillary status.

Although frozen section analysis has advantages in that that it is a rapid procedure and therefore may be used intra-operatively, it clearly has its limitations. These include:

1. Freezing artefact and hence loss of good tissue architecture and cytological detail
2. Difficulty in obtaining a good complete section consistently, especially in nodes replaced by fat (Fig. 4)
3. Difficulty in identifying small foci of tumour, particularly of the lobular type

There is concern amongst histopathologists that the sentinel node biopsy procedure will increase the workload. Even if a frozen section request becomes part of the analysis, this must be offset against time spent retrieving lymph nodes from the axillary dissection and the resources used in processing, cutting, staining and reporting the extra lymph node blocks.

Paraffin Section

Confirmatory paraffin section is done following the frozen section. Paraffin sections are assessed independently of the frozen section diagnosis. Although at present only a single paraffin section is cut after the frozen section diagnosis, it is possible that this procedure will have to be modified with the use of serial sections. However, since in total the specimen will have been examined at six levels plus a paraffin section, the use of further serial sections is unlikely to increase the yield of micrometastases substantially. Furthermore, in those cases which are negative both on frozen section and on paraffin H & E section, immunohistochemistry using a pan-cytokeratin antibody is also being used. It is anticipated that the combination of the three techniques on the sentinel node would identify more than 99 % of micrometastases. Pathology examination of the axillary dissection is currently dealt with routinely, with only a single H & E section examination of all the lymph nodes. Ideally all the lymph nodes of the axilla should also be examined at six levels and with the use of immunohistochemistry techniques; however, this is not a feasible proposition in our laboratory at present.

The final axillary status is matched up with the diagnosis from the frozen sections and the confirmatory H & E paraffin section.

Autoradiography

The distribution of radionuclide may be mapped in tissue sections by autoradiography using a radiation-sensitive film or emulsion.

Technique

Tissue biopsies are frozen and 10-µm sections cut in a cryostat at approximately –25°C; these are thaw-mounted onto gelatinised microscope slides. After drying at room temperature, tissue sections are fixed (acetone at 4°C for 30 min) before being exposed to Hyperfilm 3H (Amersham International) in X-ray cassettes overnight at room temperature. Slide-mounted tissue may be subsequently stained with haematoxylin and eosin for histology. Figure 5 shows such an autoradiograph of a sentinel node, revealing the distribution of radioactive particles along the subcapsular sinus where they are trapped by macrophages. In a study performed by Zeidman and Buss [63] it was demonstrated

that the tumour emboli are immediately trapped in the subcapsular sinus on entering the lymph node through afferent lymphatics. There is an ongoing study into the pathophysiology of radioactive colloidal particles kinetics within the lymph node in our institution.

Electron Microscopy of the Sentinel Node

Attempts to visualise the colloidal particles under conventional electron microscopy have been unsuccessful as colloidal albumin particles used to label a sentinel node are not electron dense. Figure 6a demonstrates a frozen section of a sentinel node prepared for electron microscopy. The nodal capsule and the subcapsular sinus are clearly visible. On a higher power view a macrophage is visible but the colloidal albumin is not visualised (Fig. 6b).

Future Developments

There can be little doubt that the lymph node status in the axilla is an important prognostic factor and that a certain proportion of patients who are lymph node-negative will relapse with the disease. The identification of occult lymph node metastases in this group of patients may therefore

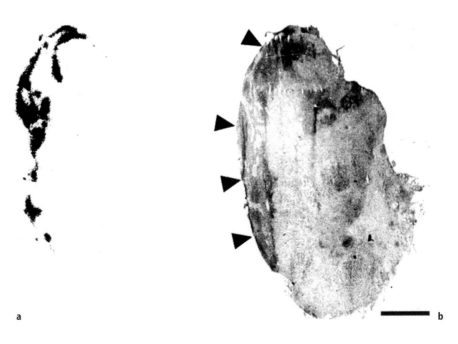

Fig. 5. **a** Autoradiograph of a sentinel node showing the distribution of radioactive particles along the subcapsular sinus. **b** Photograph of the same slide-mounted sentinel lymph node

a

b

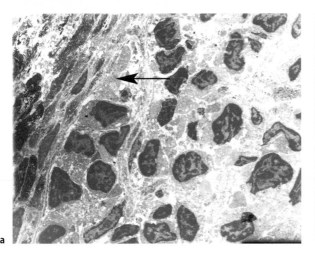

a

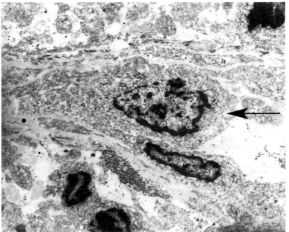

b

Fig. 6. a Electron microscopy picture of a sentinel node. The *arrow* shows the subcapsular sinus. **b** High-power view of a macrophage

be useful in planning therapy. The detection of such micrometastases with the use of serial sectioning or immunohistochemistry or molecular-based techniques is not a viable proposition for most laboratories at present. However, the developments in the use of sentinel node biopsy, which has been shown to be useful in patients with malignant melanoma, will have important implications for the management of breast cancer patients. If the ongoing studies can confirm that the investigation of the sentinel node is not only accurately predictive of the lymph node status of the axilla, but also that the false-positive rate is low, this will change the histopathological practice in the assessment of breast cancer specimens quite dramatically. It should be quite feasible for most histopathology laboratories to examine one or two lymph nodes by the use of multiple levels and even immunohistochemistry if this is all that is required for the prediction of the axillary status in most patients. Since in the majority of cases this is indeed all that would be required, it would not significantly increase the workload of the histopathology department. The use of sentinel node biopsy in the management of breast cancer patients is therefore likely to be an important advance.

References

1. Hoskins K, Weber BL. The biology of breast cancer. *Curr Opin Oncol* 1994; 6:554–559
2. Fisher B, Redmond C, Fisher ER. The contribution of recent NSABP clinical trials of primary breast cancer therapy to an understanding of tumor biology – an overview of findings. *Cancer* 1980; 46:1009–1025
3. Rosen PP, Saigo PE, Braun DW Jr, Weathers E, DePalo A. Predictors of recurrence in stage I (T1N0M0) breast carcinoma. *Ann Surg* 1981; 193:15–25
4. Fisher B, Bauer M, Wickerham DL et al. Relation of number of positive axillary nodes to the prognosis of patients with primary breast cancer. An NSABP update. *Cancer* 1983; 52:1551–1557
5. Elston CW, Ellis IO. Pathological prognostic factors in breast cancer. I. The value of histological grade in breast cancer: experience from a large study with long-term follow-up. *Histopathology* 1991; 19:403–410
6. Ellis IO, Galea M, Broughton N, Locker A, Blamey RW, Elston CW. Pathological prognostic factors in breast cancer. II. Histological type. Relationship with survival in a large study with long-term follow-up. *Histopathology* 1992; 20:479–489
7. NHSBPS Publication. *Pathology reporting in breast cancer screening.* 1995
8. Rosai J. Borderline epithelial lesions of the breast. *Am J Surg Pathol* 1991; 15:209–221
9. Sloane JP, Ellman R, Anderson TJ et al. Consistency of histopathological reporting of breast lesions detected by screening: findings of the U.K. National External Quality Assessment (EQA) Scheme. *Eur J Cancer* 1994; 30A:1414–1419
10. Saphir O, Amromin GD. Obscure axillary lymph node metastases in carcinoma of the breast. *Cancer* 1948; 1:238–241
11. Pickren JW. Significance of occult metastases. A study of breast cancer. *Cancer* 1961; 14:1266–1271
12. Huvos AG, Hutter RV, Berg JW. Significance of axillary macrometastases and micrometastases in mammary cancer. *Ann Surg* 1971; 173:44–46
13. Attiyeh FF, Jensen M, Huvos AG, Fracchia A. Axillary micrometastasis and macrometastasis in carcinoma of the breast. *Surg Gynecol Obstet* 1977; 144:839–842

14. Fisher ER, Swamidoss S, Lee CH, Rockette H, Redmond C, Fisher B. Detection and significance of occult axillary node metastases in patients with invasive breast cancer. *Cancer* 1978; 42:2025–2031

15. Sloane JP, Ormerod MG, Imrie SF, Coombes RC. The use of antisera to epithelial membrane antigen in detecting micrometastases in histological sections. *Br J Cancer* 1980; 42:392–398

16. Black RB, Roberts MM, Stewart HJ et al. The search for occult metastases in breast cancer: does it add to established staging methods? *Aust N Z J Surg* 1980; 50:574–579

17. Rosen PP, Saigo PE, Braun DW, Weathers E, Fracchia AA, Kinne DW. Axillary micro- and macrometastases in breast cancer: prognostic significance of tumor size. *Ann Surg* 1981; 194:585–591

18. Rosen PP, Saigo PE, Braun DW Jr, Beattie EJ Jr, Kinne DW. Occult axillary lymph node metastases from breast cancers with intramammary lymphatic tumor emboli. *Am J Surg Pathol* 1982; 6:639–641

19. Wilkinson EJ, Hause LL, Hoffman RG et al. Occult axillary lymph node metastases in invasive breast carcinoma: characteristics of the primary tumor and significance of the metastases. *Pathol Annu* 1982; 17:67–91

20. Wells CA, Heryet A, Brochier J, Gatter KC, Mason DY. The immunocytochemical detection of axillary micrometastases in breast cancer. *Br J Cancer* 1984; 50:193–197

21. Bussolati G, Gugliotta P, Morra I, Pietribiasi F, Berardengo E. The immunohistochemical detection of lymph node metastases from infiltrating lobular carcinoma of the breast. *Br J Cancer* 1986; 54:631–636

22. Byrne J, Waldron R, McAvinchey D, Dervan P. The use of monoclonal antibodies for the histopathological detection of mammary axillary micrometastases. *Eur J Surg Oncol* 1987; 13:409–411

23. Trojani M, de Mascarel I, Bonichon F, Coindre JM, Delsol G. Micrometastases to axillary lymph nodes from carcinoma of breast: detection by immunohistochemistry and prognostic significance. *Br J Cancer* 1987; 55:303–306

24. Friedman S, Bertin F, Mouriesse H et al. Importance of tumor cells in axillary node sinus margins ('clandestine' metastases) discovered by serial sectioning in operable breast carcinoma. *Acta Oncol* 1988; 27:483–487

25. Berry N, Jones DB, Marshall R, Smallwood J, Taylor I. Comparison of the detection of breast carcinoma metastases by routine histological diagnosis and by immunohistochemical staining. *Eur Surg Res* 1988; 20:225–232

26. Apostolikas N, Petraki C, Agnantis NJ. The reliability of histologically negative axillary lymph nodes in breast cancer. Preliminary report. *Pathol Res Pract* 1988; 184:35–38

27. Sedmak DD, Meineke TA, Knechtges DS. Detection of metastatic breast carcinoma with monoclonal antibodies to cytokeratins [see comments]. *Arch Pathol Lab Med* 1989; 113:786–789

28. Raymond WA, Leong AS. Immunoperoxidase staining in the detection of lymph node metastases in stage I breast cancer. *Pathology* 1989; 21:11–15

29. Ludwig Breast Cancer Study Group. Prognostic importance of occult axillary lymph node micrometastases from breast cancers. International (Ludwig) Breast Cancer Study Group. *Lancet* 1990; 335:1565–1568

30. Springall RJ, Rytina E, Millis RR. Incidence and significance of micrometastases in axillary lymph nodes detected by immunohistochemical techniques. *J Pathol* 1990: 174 A

31. Galea MH, Athanassiou E, Bell J et al. Occult regional lymph node metastases from breast carcinoma: immunohistological detection with antibodies CAM 5.2 and NCRC-11. *J Pathol* 1991; 165:221–227

32. Chen ZL, Wen DR, Coulson WF, Giuliano AE, Cochran AJ. Occult metastases in the axillary lymph nodes of patients with breast cancer node negative by clinical and histologic examination and conventional histology. *Dis Markers* 1991; 9:239–248

33. Neville AM. Breast cancer micrometastases in lymph nodes and bone marrow are prognostically important. *Ann Oncol* 1991; 2:13–14

34. Byrne J, Horgan PG, England S, Callaghan J, Given HF. A preliminary report on the usefulness of monoclonal antibodies to CA 15-3 and MCA in the detection of micrometastases in axillary lymph nodes draining primary breast carcinoma. *Eur J Cancer* 1992 ; 28:658–660

35. de Mascarel I, Bonichon F, Coindre JM, Trojani M. Prognostic significance of breast cancer axillary lymph node micrometastases assessed by two special techniques: re-evaluation with longer follow-up. *Br J Cancer* 1992; 66:523–527

36. Nasser IA, Lee AK, Bosari S, Saganich R, Heatley G, Silverman ML. Occult axillary lymph node metastases in "node-negative" breast carcinoma. *Hum Pathol* 1993; 24:950–957

37. Hainsworth PJ, Tjandra JJ, Stillwell RG et al. Detection and significance of occult metastases in node-negative breast cancer. *Br J Surg* 1993; 80:459–463

38. Clayton F, Hopkins CL. Pathologic correlates of prognosis in lymph node-positive breast carcinomas. *Cancer* 1993; 71:1780–1790

39. Elson CE, Kufe D, Johnston WW. Immunohistochemical detection and significance of axillary lymph node micrometastases in breast carcinoma. A study of 97 cases. *Anal Quant Cytol Histol* 1993; 15:171–178

40. McGuckin MA, Cummings MC, Walsh MD, Hohn BG, Bennett IC, Wright RG. Occult axillary node metastases in breast cancer: their detection and prognostic significance. *Br J Cancer* 1996; 73:88–95

41. Mori M, Mimori K, Inoue H et al. Detection of cancer micrometastases in lymph nodes by reverse transcriptase-polymerase chain reaction. *Cancer Res* 1995; 55:3417–3420

42. Mori M, Mimori K, Ueo H et al. Molecular detection of circulating solid carcinoma cells in the peripheral blood: the concept of early systemic disease. *Int J Cancer* 1996; 68:739–743

43. Mori M, Mimori K, Ueo H et al. Clinical significance of molecular detection of carcinoma cells in lymph nodes and peripheral blood by reverse transcription-polymerase chain reaction in patients with gastrointestinal or breast carcinomas. *J Clin Oncol* 1998; 16:128–132

44. Noguchi S, Aihara T, Motomura K, Inaji H, Imaoka S, Koyama H. Histologic characteristics of breast cancers with occult lymph node metastases detected by keratin 19 mRNA reverse transcriptase-polymerase chain reaction. *Cancer* 1996; 78:1235–1240

45. Noguchi S, Aihara T, Motomura K, Inaji H, Imaoka S, Koyama H. Detection of breast cancer micrometastases in axillary lymph nodes by means of reverse transcriptase-polymerase chain reaction. Comparison between MUC 1 mRNA and keratin 19 mRNA amplification. *Am J Pathol* 1996; 148:649–656

46. Schoenfeld A, Luqmani Y, Smith D et al. Detection of breast cancer micrometastases in axillary lymph nodes by using polymerase chain reaction. *Cancer Res* 1994; 54: 2986–2990

47. Bostick PJ, Chatterjee S, Chi DD et al. Limitations of specific reverse-transcriptase polymerase chain reaction markers in the detection of metastases in the lymph nodes and blood of breast cancer patients. *J Clin Oncol* 1998; 16: 2632–2640

48. Giuliano AE, Jones RC, Brennan M, Statman R. Sentinel lymphadenectomy in breast cancer. *J Clin Oncol* 1997; 15:2345–2350

49. Giuliano AE, Kirgan DM, Guenther JM, Morton DL. Lymphatic mapping and sentinel lymphadenectomy for breast cancer [see comments]. *Ann Surg* 1994; 220:391–398; discussion 398–401

50. Borgstein PJ, Meijer S, Pijpers R. Intradermal blue dye to identify sentinel lymph-node in breast cancer. *Lancet* 1997; 349:1668–1669

51. Borgstein PJ, Pijpers R, Comans EF, van Diest PJ, Boom RP, Meijer S. Sentinel lymph node biopsy in breast cancer: guidelines and pitfalls of lymphoscintigraphy and gamma probe detection. *J Am Coll Surg* 1998; 186:275–283

52. Crossin JA, Johnson AC, Stewart PB, Turner WW Jr. Gamma-probe-guided resection of the sentinel lymph node in breast cancer. *Am Surg* 1998; 64:666–668; discussion 669

53. Barnwell JM, Arredondo MA, Kollmorgen D et al. Sentinel node biopsy in breast cancer. *Ann Surg Oncol* 1998; 5: 126–130

54. Guenther JM, Krishnamoorthy M, Tan LR. Sentinel lymphadenectomy for breast cancer in a community managed care setting. *Cancer J Sci Am* 1997; 3:336–340

55. Alex JC, Krag DN. The gamma-probe-guided resection of radiolabeled primary lymph nodes. *Surg Oncol Clin North Am* 1996; 5:33–41

56. Veronesi U, Paganelli G, Galimberti V et al. Sentinel-node biopsy to avoid axillary dissection in breast cancer with clinically negative lymph-nodes. *Lancet* 1997; 349: 1864–1867

57. Turner RR, Ollila DW, Krasne DL, Giuliano AE. Histopathologic validation of the sentinel lymph node hypothesis for breast carcinoma. *Ann Surg* 1997; 226:271–276; discussion 276–278

58. Krag D, Weaver D, Ashikaga T et al. The sentinel node in breast cancer – a multicenter validation study. *N Engl J Med* 1998; 339:941–946

59. O'Hea BJ, Hill AD, El-Shirbiny AM et al. Sentinel lymph node biopsy in breast cancer: initial experience at Memorial Sloan-Kettering Cancer Center. *J Am Coll Surg* 1998; 186:423–427

60. Dale PS, Williams JTT. Axillary staging utilizing selective sentinel lymphadenectomy for patients with invasive breast carcinoma. *Am Surg* 1998; 64:28–31; discussion 32

61. Albertini JJ, Lyman GH, Cox C et al. Lymphatic mapping and sentinel node biopsy in the patient with breast cancer. *JAMA* 1996; 276:1818–1822

62. Belli F, Lenisa L, Clemente C et al. Sentinel node biopsy and selective dissection for melanoma nodal metastases. *Tumori* 1998; 84:24–28

63. Zeidman I, Buss JM. Experimental studies on the spread of cancer in lymphatic system – Effectiveness of the lymph node as a barrier to the passage of embolic tumour cells. *Cancer Res* 1954; 14:403–405

CHAPTER 10

Cytology of the Sentinel Node

GABRIJELA KOCJAN

Introduction

Cytological investigation of sentinel nodes is performed by means of peri-operative imprints or fine-needle aspiration (FNA) samples. Neither of the techniques is new. Indeed, imprint cytology is one of the oldest methods in cytopathology and is probably underutilised at present [1, 2]. Its decline is thought to be associated with the rise of FNA cytology. FNA cytology has wider applications. FNA samples can be taken pre-operatively from multiple sites. Intra-operatively, both imprint and FNA preparations from fresh (unfixed) lymph nodes serve to provide diagnostic information before the permanent tissue sections are available [3]. The imprint method has proven useful in the intra-operative staging of lymphadenopathy and has been used as an alternative to frozen section [4–6].

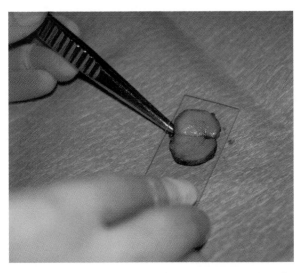

Fig. 1. Preparation of cytological imprint preparations by touching of glass slides with the freshly cut surface of the lymph node

Preparation of Material

After excision, lymph nodes are halved and the cut surface touched onto glass slides, resulting in cell imprints (Fig. 1). These are stained with rapid cytological stain (RAL 555, Cell Path, UK), enabling reading of the slides within 3 min. FNA samples are taken from the same nodes by means of a 23-G needle, a 20-ml syringe and a syringe holder (Cameco) (Fig. 2). Material is spread onto glass slides and air dried. Some of the material from both imprints and FNA smears is left for special stains and immunocytochemistry that can be performed within 15 min or later. Slides are examined under the light microscope. Imprint cytology from lymph nodes provides excellent cytological detail.

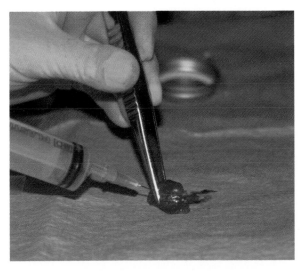

Fig. 2. Fine-needle aspiration of the excised sentinel node by using a 23-G needle, a 20-ml syringe and a syringe holder. Smears are air dried and stained with rapid stain

Microscopic Findings

Typical microscopic findings from a reactive sentinel node imprint stained with rapid stains show numerous lymphoid cells. These appear in large aggregates (Fig. 3) and single cells including a variety of follicle centre cells (Fig. 4). In cases where patent blue dye has been applied, occasional tingible body macrophages may contain the blue dye granules (Fig. 5).

In cases of metastatic disease large aggregates of epithelial cells are seen (Fig. 6). These cells are much larger than lymphoid cells and show cytological features of malignancy (Fig. 7a). Immuno-

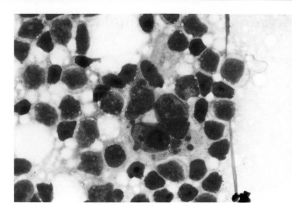

Fig. 5. High-power view of the tingible body macrophage containing blue pigment, presumably from the contrast medium. MGG × 600, oil immersion

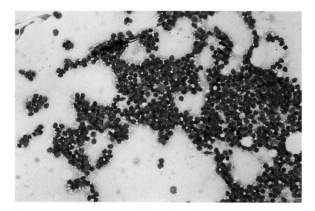

Fig. 3. Low-power view of lymph node imprint. Numerous lymphoid cells are present in a trabecular pattern surrounding the globules of fat. MGG, × 100

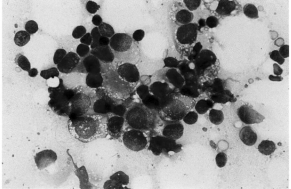

Fig. 6. Aggregate of malignant epithelial cells in a lymph node imprint. Epithelial cells are larger than lymphocytes and show cytological features of malignancy. MGG, × 400

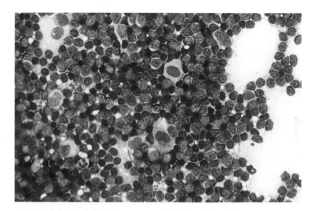

Fig. 4. Sentinel node imprint cytology. Numerous lymphoid cells and tingible body macrophages suggest reactive hyperplasia only. No evidence of metastatic tumour. MGG, × 200, oil immersion

cytochemical investigation shows these cells to be strongly positive for cytokeratin, thus confirming metastatic disease (Fig. 7b).

The Role of Sentinel Node Imprint Cytology in Management, and Possible Pitfalls

Lymphatic mapping of axillary lymph nodes is technically feasible and reliably identifies sentinel nodes in most cases, the overall success being maximised when blue dye and radioisotope techniques are used together [7]. The potential role of intra-operative imprint cytology of resected axillary nodes in patients with breast carcinoma

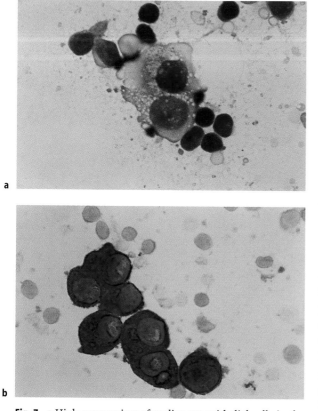

Fig. 7. a High-power view of malignant epithelial cells in the lymph node imprint. These show irregular nuclei and prominent nucleoli. MGG, × 600, oil immersion. **b** Immunocytochemical markers for cytokeratin confirm the epithelial nature of large cells and also confirm metastases. MNF 116, APAAP, × 600, oil immersion

undergoing axillary clearance was studied by Fisher et al. [8]. Among 50 patients with axillary clearance, 21 of whom had histologically confirmed metastatic disease, intra-operative imprint cytology detected 18/21 positive nodes. It was established that, should the technique of imprint cytology have been used intra-operatively, 29 out of 50 patients would have avoided the operation, one would have had to have undergone extended axillary surgery and two would not have received further axillary surgery. According to O'Hea et al. the diagnostic accuracy of sentinel nodes in predicting metastatic disease in the axilla is 95% (these authors obtained false-negative results in 3/55 patients in whom sentinel nodes were identified) [7]. A negative sentinel node biopsy may eliminate the need for axillary lymph node dissection for select women with breast cancer [9].

The results of peri-operative imprint cytology of lymph nodes in resections of lung cancer and mediastinum show a similar high accuracy of 97.3% – 99.2% and a sensitivity of 96.6% – 100% [10, 11]. Compared with frozen histological section, imprint cytology is more rapid (average 2 min versus 11 min) and allows more extensive sampling of the specimen [11].

The potential pitfalls of sentinel node imprint cytology are of two kinds: those due to technical preparation and those due to interpretation. The preparation of imprints, although technically not very demanding and producing an abundance of cells, creates layers of various cell thickness and an unpredictable pattern of cell distribution on the slide. Some of the thicker cell layers take longer to air dry (and are therefore subject to drying artefacts) and make it difficult for the rapid stains to penetrate; they then appear pale on screening and on low power may appear to be non-lymphoid (Fig. 8). We found spreading of the smears from an FNA by an experienced hand, to be technically superior to imprints, producing a monolayer of cells of similar density. The drawback of the latter method is that it is operator dependent. The interpretation pitfalls are illustrated by the presence of a single malignant cell in a sea of lymphocytes (Fig. 9 a), comparable to the appearance of follicular dendritic cells from a reactive lymph node (Fig. 9 b).

In a study of 109 sentinel node imprints from 86 patients, 26 of which harboured micrometastases, Ahmad et al. found that 14 were not detected

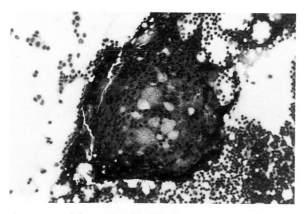

Fig. 8. One of the potential pitfalls in imprint cytology is the presence of large aggregates of lymphoid cells, which may appear to be epithelial. RAL, × 100

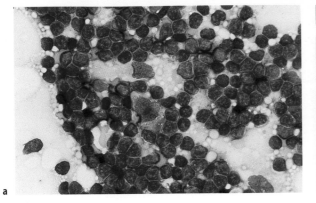
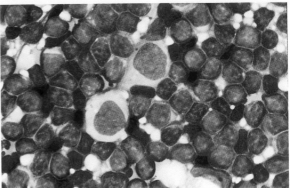

a

b

Fig. 9. a Another pitfall in the imprint cytology may be the presence of single malignant cells, as illustrated in this field where a single malignant cell is present in the centre and can be mistaken for follicular dendritic cells × 400. **b** Higher power view × 600

by imprint cytology and three were not detected by permanent histopathology [12]. They found that immunocytochemistry performed on cytological preparations detected micrometastases in 23 out of 26 cases, thus upstaging the nodal status previously identified on either imprint cytology or histology. They concluded that sentinel node imprints and histology findings can be improved by the use of intra-operative immunocytochemistry (anticytokeratin). The reliance on immunocytochemistry may be the reason for the relatively poor diagnostic accuracy of imprint cytology in this series. The presence of false-positive as well as false-negative results even in a series with 94.5 % overall diagnostic accuracy of imprint cytology of lymph nodes in patients with breast neoplasms implies a need for caution with interpreting [13]. Even present-day immunocytochemistry, shown to be superior to morphological assessment on the basis of routine staining alone, can be misleading. The choice of immunocytochemical markers and knowledge of their cross-reaction with normal cells are important. The case depicted in Fig. 10 illustrates how a commonly used anticytokeratin antibody stains some normal constituents of the lymph node, which can be recognised in most instances by their morphology (long cytoplasmic processes). The study of interobserver agreement and diagnostic accuracy of lymph node imprint cytodiagnosis found it to have a 91.2 % positive predictive value

for detection of secondary malignancy. The values were lower for diagnosis of lymphomas and reactive change [14].

Conclusion

The technique of sentinel node resection combined with intra-operative lymph node imprint cytology may be useful in reducing the morbidity of breast cancer surgery without increasing the risk of locoregional or distant recurrence. Imprint cytology may be used as an adjunct to or substitute for frozen section histology. Intra-operative immunocytochemistry may be used to improve the diagnostic accuracy of this method. Both the surgeon and the pathologist should be aware of the potential pitfalls in diagnosis.

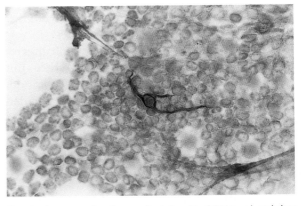

Fig. 10. An example of an anticytokeratin (CAM 5.2) staining follicular dendritic cells (red cells with long processes) which are part of the reactive lymph node cell population but can be mistaken for metastatic cells. APAAP, × 400

References

1. Ultmann JE, Koprowska I, Engle RL. A cytological study of lymph node imprints. *Cancer* 1958; 11:507–524
2. Aust R, Stahle J, Stenkvist B. The imprint method for the cytodiagnosis of lymphadenopathies and of tumours of the head and neck. *Acta Cytol* 1971; 15:123–127
3. Koo CH, Rappaport H, Sheibani K, Pengalis GA, Nathwani BN, Winberg CD. Imprint cytology of non-Hodgkin's lymphomas based on a study of 212 immunologically characterised cases: correlation of touch imprints with tissue sections. *Hum Pathol* 1989; 20:1–137
4. Ghandur-Mnaymneh L, Paz J. The use of touch preparations (tissue imprints) in the rapid intraoperative diagnosis of metastatic lymph node disease in cancer staging procedures. *Cancer* 1985; 56:339–344
5. Gentry JF. Pelvic lymph node metastases in prostatic cancer. The value of touch imprint cytology. *Am J Surg Pathol* 1986; 10:718–727
6. Bhabra K, Goulden RG, Peel KR. Intra-operative diagnosis of lymph node metastases in gynaecological practice using imprint cytology. *Eur J Gynaecol Oncol* 1989; 10:117–124
7. O'Hea BJ, Hill AD, El Shirbiny AM, Rosen PP, Coit DG, Borgen PI, Cody HS. Sentinel lymph node biopsy in breast cancer: initial experience at Memorial Sloan-Kettering Cancer Center. *J Am Coll Surg* 1988; 186:423–427
8. Fisher CJ, Boyle S, Burke M, Price AB. Intraoperative assessment of nodal status in the selection of patients with breast cancer for axillary clearance. *Br J Surg* 1993; 80:457–458
9. Barnwell JM, Arredondo MA, Kollmorgen D, Gibbs JF, Lamonica D, Carson W, Zhang P, Winston J, Edge SB. Sentinel node biopsy in breast cancer. *Ann Surg Oncol* 1998; 5:126–130
10. Tsukada H, Akaogi E, Ogawa I et al. Imprint cytodiagnosis of lymph node metastasis in resected lung cancer. *Nippon Kyobu Shikkan Gakkai Zasshi* 1992; 30:91–94
11. Clarke MR, Landreanau RJ, Borochowitz D. Intraoperative imprint cytology for evaluation of mediastinal lymphadenopathy. *Ann Thorac Surg* 1994; 57:1206–1210
12. Ahmad N, Ku NNN, Nicosia SV, Smith PV, Muro Cacho CA, Livingston S, Reintgen DS, Cox CE. Evaluation of sentinel lymph node imprints in breast cancer: role of intraoperative cytokeratin immunostaining in breast cancer staging. *Acta Cytol* 1998; 42:1218
13. Molyneux AJ, Atanoos RL, Coghill SB. The value of lymph node imprint cytodiagnosis: an assessment of interobserver agreement and diagnostic accuracy. *Cytopathology* 1997; 8:256–264
14. Heidenreich JK, Schussler J, Borner P, Dehnhard F, Deicher H, Kalden J, Peter HH. Imprint cytology of axillary lymph nodes in breast neoplasms for intraoperative rapid diagnosis. *Fortschr Med* 1978; 96:1366–1368

Clinical Case Material

There is no substitute for experience, and illustrations and descriptions of clinical case material can only be considered as a guide to practice. Nevertheless, it is possible to use such material to draw the attention of the interested reader to a number of items which may contribute to faster appreciation of the variety and peculiarities that will be encountered in the performance of the sentinel node detection procedure.

Here we present a selection of cases from our routine experience. We hope that these are interesting and helpful, and that they will complement the other data and information provided in this book. This case selection is not intended to be all-inclusive or comprehensive but it will offer a reasonable sample of the material one encounters in a typical hospital environment. Each clinical case has a teaching point. A short history introduces the clinical problem and a selection of image data completes the descriptive material. The data are displayed on two juxtaposed pages to assist the reader in readily absorbing the information.

Mucinous Breast Carcinoma

A 79-year-old female presented with a lump in the left breast. On examination, there was a 2-cm mobile lump in the upper outer quadrant of the breast. There was no clinical evidence of axillary node involvement. Pre-operative investigation confirmed the diagnosis of mucinous carcinoma. Considering the patient's age and the good prognosis of the tumour, she underwent wide local excision and sentinel node biopsy only.

Operative Findings

At operation, the site of the sentinel node was confirmed with Neoprobe 1500 prior to incision. Through a 2.5-cm incision, the axilla was explored and with a 14-mm probe; the sentinel node was easily localised. The patient underwent wide local excision of the primary tumour.

Dynamic Imaging

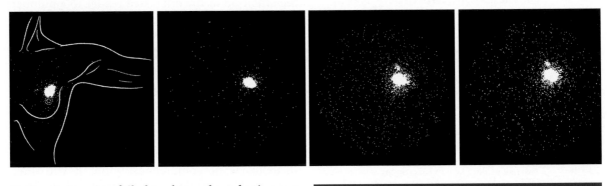

Dynamic imaging failed to show a lymphatic tract and towards the end of dynamic acquisition a focal area of radioactivity uptake was evident very close to the injection site.

Histology

Histology confirmed a grade 1 mucinous carcinoma measuring 2 cm in its maximum dimension. The sentinel node was free of metastatic tumour on H & E staining and immunohistochemistry. Oestrogen receptor status was positive.

Static Imaging

Prior to static acquisition, the breast was retracted downwards and medially to prevent the masking of the sentinel node from the injection site. An area of increased focal uptake was then clearly demonstrated in the axilla. The overlying skin was marked.

Teaching Point

This case demonstrates that in elderly patients with a good-prognosis early breast carcinoma, sentinel node biopsy can be considered. This may avoid morbidity associated with an axillary node clearance in a low-risk case.

Static Imaging

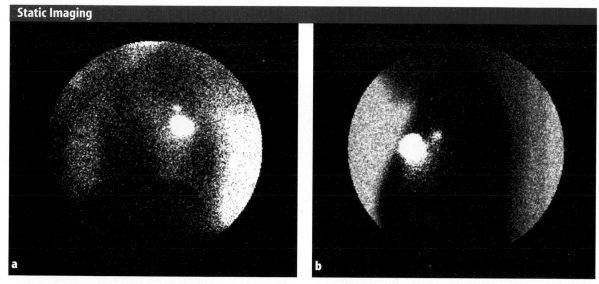

a Anterior-oblique view
b Lateral view

Histology

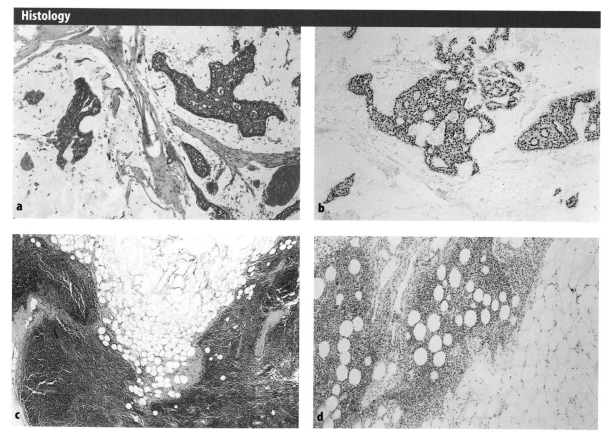

a Grade-1 mucinous carcinoma (H & E)
b Positive oestrogen receptor (ER Positive)
c The sentinel node free of metastatic tumour (H & E)
d Negative sentinel node (MNF 116)

Lobular Breast Carcinoma

A 56-year-old female presented with a large mass in her left breast. She had undergone modified radical mastectomy 7 years previously for invasive lobular carcinoma of the right breast. On examination, there was a large central breast lump. There was no clinical evidence of axillary lymph node involvement.

Investigation confirmed the diagnosis of invasive lobular carcinoma. Screening investigations for distant metastasis, including bone scan, chest X-ray and liver function tests were negative. The patient consented for mastectomy and sentinel node biopsy only, owing to her unpleasant experience with axillary clearance on the other side in the past.

Operative Findings

The axilla was explored through the mastectomy incision. A hot lymph mode was evident with Neoprobe 1500 that had not taken up the blue dye.

Histology

Histology of the primary tumour confirmed the diagnosis of grade 1 invasive lobular carcinoma on the mastectomy specimen. The sentinel node was heavily replaced with metastatic lobular carcinoma. Oestrogen receptor status was strongly positive.

Dynamic Imaging

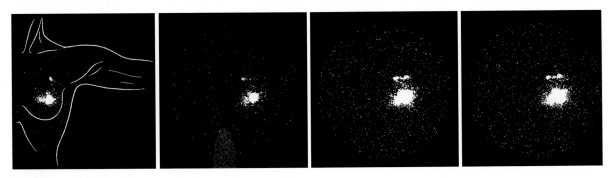

Dynamic imaging revealed a faint lymphatic tract with two areas of increased focal activity.

Static Imaging

Static imaging confirmed two areas of increased uptake on the anterior-oblique and the lateral views.

Teaching Point

Sentinel node biopsy showed evidence of metastatic lobular carcinoma. On this basis, the patient was recommended to have axillary node dissection and adjuvant chemotherapy.

Static Imaging

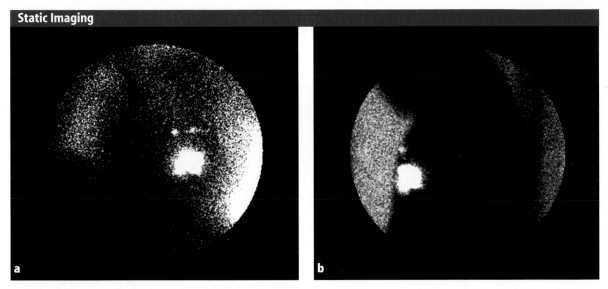

a Anterior-oblique view
b Lateral view

Histology

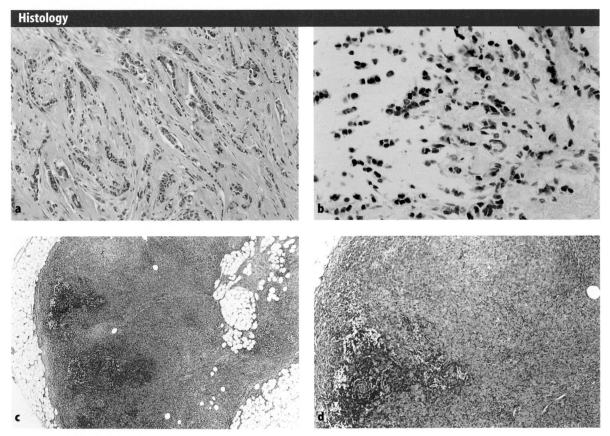

a Grade-1 invasive lobular carcinoma (H & E)
b Strongly positive oestrogen receptor (ER Positive)
c Sentinel node completely replaced with metastatic lobular carcinoma (H & E)
d High power view of the SLN showing complete replacement with metastatic carcinoma (H & E)

Papillary Carcinoma of the Breast

An 86-year-old female presented with a 6-week history of lump in the left breast. She was walking with two sticks as a result of a recent bilateral patellar fracture. She also suffered from a very stiff left shoulder. On examination, there was a 4-cm lump in the upper outer quadrant of the left breast and no palpable axillary lymph nodes. Investigations confirmed the diagnosis of breast cancer and the patient opted to have a mastectomy and sentinel node biopsy as she did not want to go through with postoperative radiotherapy.

Lymphoscintigraphy

Lymphoscintigraphy was performed by injecting 15 MBq of ^{99m}Tc-colloidal albumin (Albures) at the site of the tumour. Dynamic acquisition was not performed due to the patient's shoulder problem.

Static Imaging

Static imaging confirmed presence of a sentinel node, close to the injection site in the axillary tail of the breast.

Operative Findings

At operation the sentinel node was found in the axillary tail, with the Neoprobe 1500. It was biopsied through the mastectomy incision.

Histology

Histology revealed at 3 cm grade 1 invasive papillary carcinoma with some papillary ductal carcinoma in situ. Oestrogen receptor status was positive and the sentinel node was free of metastasis on H & E staining and immunohistochemistry.

Static Imaging

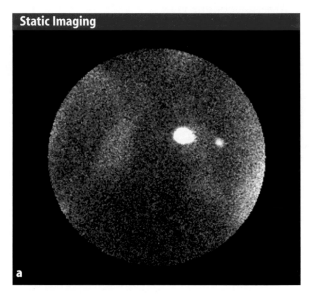

a Anterior-oblique view

Teaching Point

Sentinel node biopsy can be considered in elderly breast cancer patients with shoulder stiffness due to arthritis. In this case, lymphoscintigraphy was very helpful in revealing the sentinel node in an unusual position in the axillary tail of the breast, which would have been missed on routine axillary clearance.

Static Imaging

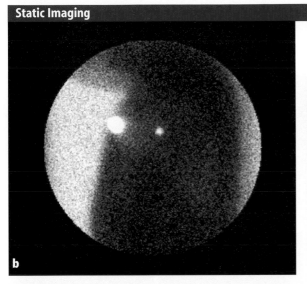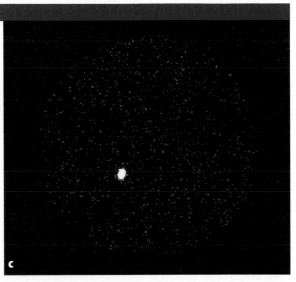

b Lateral view
c Ex-vivo image of the sentinel node after biopsy

Histology

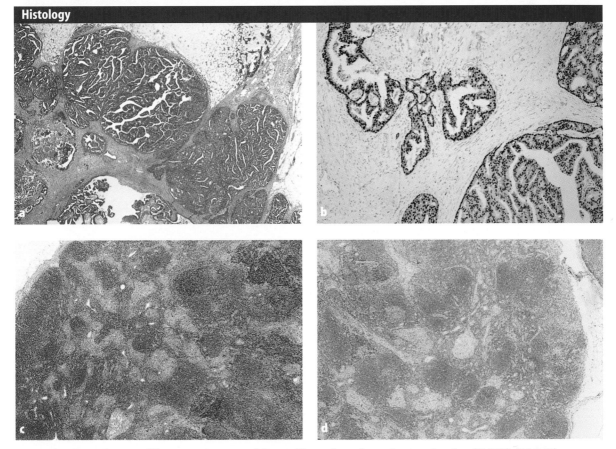

a Grade-1 invasive papillary carcinoma with papillary ductal carcinoma in-situ (DCIS) (H & E)
b Positive oestrogen receptor staining (ER Positive)
c Negative sentinel node (H & E)
d Negative sentinel node (MNF 116)

Advanced, Multifocal Breast Carcinoma

A 76-year-old female presented with a large lump in her left breast. On examination she had a 6.5-cm lump in the upper inner quadrant of the left breast with peau d'orange. There were no palpable axillary lymph nodes. A mammogram confirmed the diagnosis of breast cancer and also revealed that the tumour was multifocal.

Dynamic Imaging

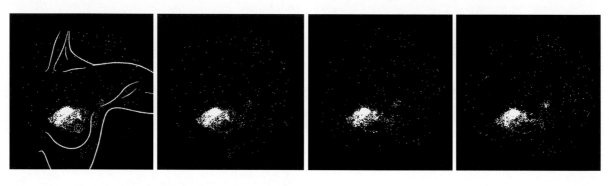

Dynamic imaging revealed several lymphatic tracts with slow progression of the tracer. A focal area of accumulation was noted in the axilla 17 min after tracer administration and this was confirmed by a static acquisition with the gamma camera.

Static Imaging

A single hot spot in the axilla was seen and the overlying skin was marked with an indelible pen.

Operative Findings

At operation, 2 ml of patent blue dye was injected subdermally. At exploration of the axilla, no blue lymph node was found. With the Neoprobe 1500 gamma detection probe, a hot node was detected which was biopsied and sent separately for histological examination. This was followed by axillary clearance.

Histology

Histology showed a multifocal grade 2 invasive ductal carcinoma. The sentinel node did not contain any metastatic deposits as judged by H & E staining and immunohistochemistry. Three of the other axillary non-sentinel nodes did show involvement by metastasis.

Teaching Point

Sentinel node biopsy should not be performed in multifocal breast tumours as this can lead to a false-negative histology result.

Mammography

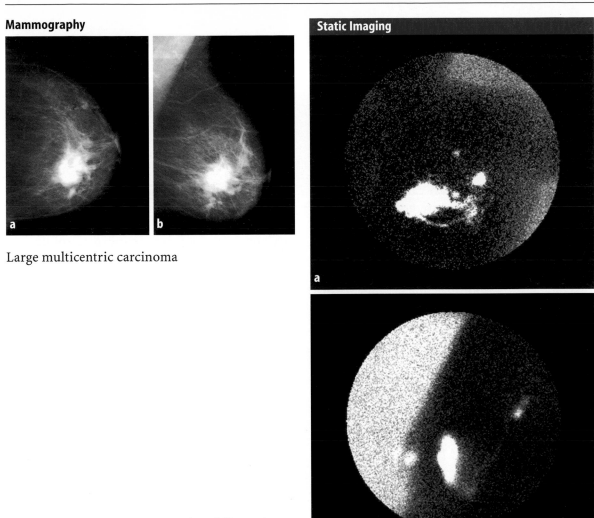

Large multicentric carcinoma

Static Imaging

Anterior-oblique view **a**
Lateral view **b**

Histology

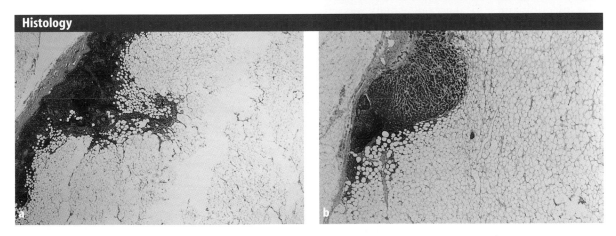

a Sentinel node not involved with cancer and replaced by fat (H & E)
b Non-sentinel node involved with cancer and replaced by fat (H & E)

Non-palpable Breast Carcinoma

A 60-year-old female was referred with a small lesion in the left breast lateral to the nipple which had been detected on a breast screening program. On examination, there was no palpable breast lump and examination of the axilla was unremarkable. Ultrasound-guided cytology confirmed the diagnosis of invasive breast carcinoma. The patient underwent pre-operative needle localisation of the lesion.

Lymphoscintigraphy
The needle that was left in situ for localisation of the lesion was used for injection of radiopharmaceutical for lymphoscintigraphy.

Operative Findings
The sentinel node was easily localised with the Neoprobe 1500. It was biopsied and sent for histology. The patient underwent wide local excision and axillary clearance.

Histology

Histology revealed a 5-mm grade 1 invasive ductal carcinoma with positive oestrogen receptors. The sentinel node was free of tumour and none of the nine other axillary lymph nodes contained metastatic cancer.

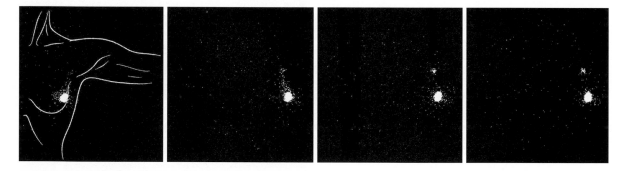

Dynamic Imaging
Dynamic imaging revealed a lymphatic tract soon after injection and a focal area of activity was evident 7 min after injection.

Static Imaging

Static imaging confirmed the presence of a sentinel node in the axillary tail which was marked on the skin.

Teaching Point

Breast cancers detected by a screening program are ideal for sentinel node biopsy. Radiopharmaceutical can be injected during needle localisation of the lesion under ultrasound or mammographic control. This case demonstrates how the sentinel node can correctly predict the status of the other axillary lymph nodes in early breast cancer.

Static Imaging

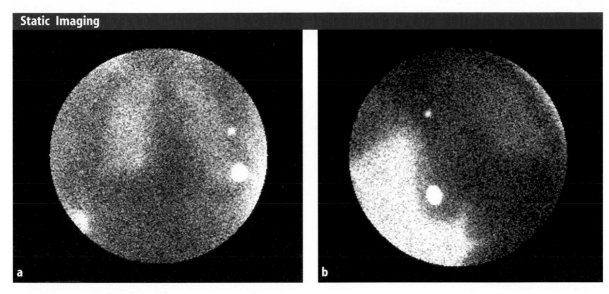

a Left anterior-oblique view
b Lateral view, hanging breast postion

Histology

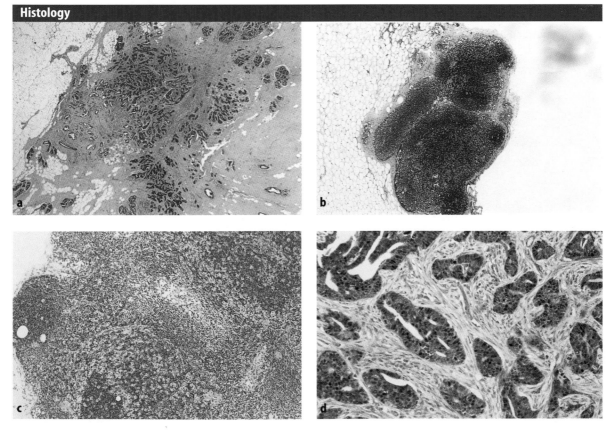

a Grade-1 invasive ductal carcinoma (H & E)
b The sentinel node free of tumour (H & E)
c Negative immunohistochemistry (MNF 116)
d Positive oestrogen receptors (ER Positive)

Non-palpable Lower Inner Quadrant Breast Carcinoma

A 70-year-old asymptomatic female was referred with a suspicious lesion in the left breast, detected on screening mammography. On examination of the breast there was no palpable lump and axillary examination did not reveal any palpable lymph nodes. Mammography showed a small suspicious mass in the lower inner quadrant and fine-needle cytology confirmed the diagnosis of breast cancer.

Lymphoscintigraphy

Lymphoscintigraphy was performed by subdermal injection of 10 MBq of ^{99cm}Tc-Albures. As the lesion was superficial, the overlying skin was marked by the radiologist for the purpose of injection.

Dynamic Imaging

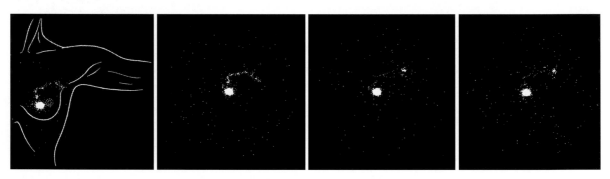

Dynamic imaging revealed rapid progression of the tracer towards the axilla, with a lymphatic tract clearly visible.

Static Imaging

Static imaging confirmed the presence of an area of increased focal radioactivity in the lower axilla.

Operative Findings

The sentinel node was identified without any difficulty with the Neoprobe 1500. This was biopsied and the patient underwent axillary node clearance and wide local excision of the primary carcinoma.

Histology

Sections of breast showed a grade 1 invasive ductal carcinoma. Histology of the sentinel node revealed no evidence of metastatic carcinoma on H & E staining or immunohistochemistry. The remaining 11 axillary lymph nodes were free of tumour.

Teaching Point

In superficial non-palpable breast carcinoma, the skin overlying the primary lesion can be marked under image guidance by the radiologist to facilitate the injection of the radiopharmaceutical (see Chap. 5, Fig. 8).

Static Imaging

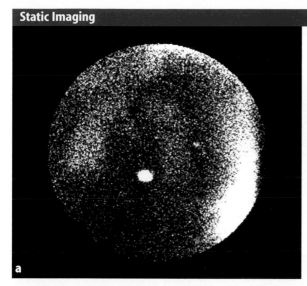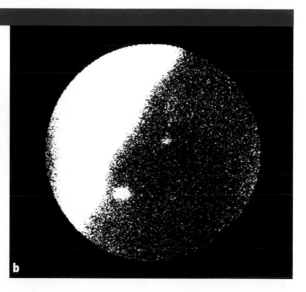

a Anterior-oblique view
b Lateral view

Histology

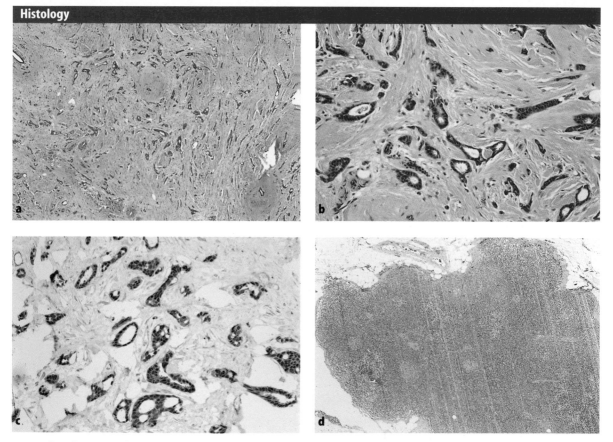

a Grade-1 invasive ductal carcinoma (H & E)
b High power view of the tumour showing tubule formation (H & E)
c Oestrogen receptor positive (ER Positive)
d Frozen section of sentinel node. No evidence of metastatic carcinoma (H & E)

Lower Outer Quadrant Lesion and Previous Breast Surgery

A 42-year-old female presented with a 6-week history of a lump in the lower outer quadrant of the right breast. She had had excision of a benign lump from the upper outer quadrant of the same breast 11 months previously. On examination there was an ill-defined nodular area in the lower outer quadrant of right breast which turned out to be a breast carcinoma.

Dynamic Imaging

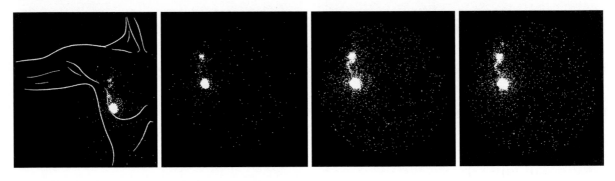

Dynamic imaging demonstrated a rapid focal accumulation of the radiopharmaceutical in the right axilla.

Static Imaging

On static imaging two areas of focal uptake were seen, one very hot spot and the other a weak one higher up.

Operative Findings

On exploring the axilla, a very hot lymph node was detected at level 1 which was also blue. As we knew from scintigraphic images about the presence of the second node, on re-applying the probe a less active node was found higher up, at level 2 in the axilla.

Histology

Histology revealed a grade 3 invasive ductal carcinoma with high-grade DCIS. The weaker sentinel node was completely replaced with metastatic carcinoma whilst the very hot and blue node was free of tumour. There were no micrometastases on immunohistochemistry. Nineteen other lymph nodes from 24 nodes dissected had metastatic cancer.

Teaching Point

Lymphoscintigraphy is important in the pre-operative localisation of the sentinel node and intra-operatively it is good practice to re-apply the gamma detection probe to look for any residual activity from other radioactive nodes, after resection of the sentinel node.

Static Imaging

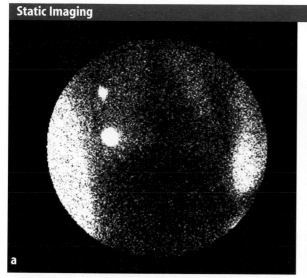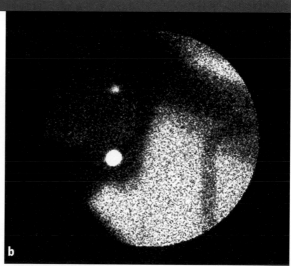

a Right anterior-oblique view
b Lateral view, hanging breast position

Histology

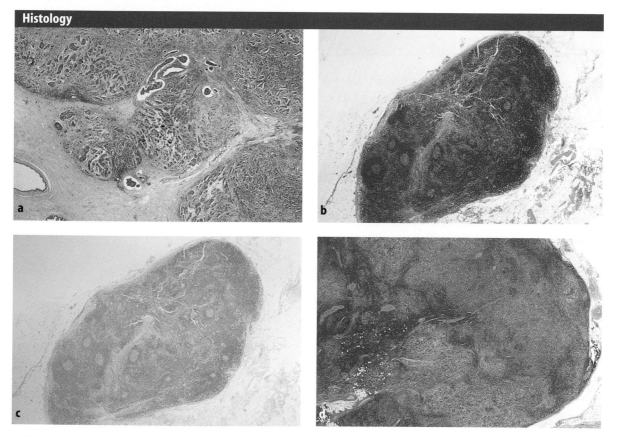

a Grade-3 invasive ductal carcinoma with high grade DCIS (H & E)
b The very hot sentinel node free of metastatic tumour (H & E)
c Negative immunohistochemistry (MNF 116)
d The weaker sentinel node completely replaced with metastatic carcinoma (H & E)

Central Breast Carcinoma

A 76-year-old female presented with a lump in her right breast. On examination, there was a 3.5-cm lump located in the retroareolar region behind the nipple. There was no clinical evidence of axillary node involvement. Investigations including core-cut biopsy confirmed the diagnosis of lobular breast carcinoma.

Dynamic Imaging

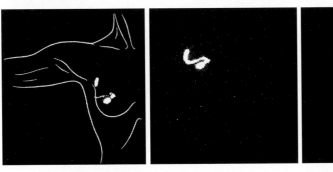 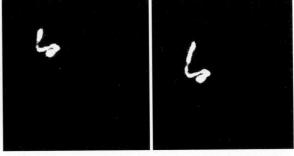

Dynamic imaging showed a very rapid transit of radioactive tracer towards the axilla. There was a very prominent lymphatic tract leading to an area of increased focal activity.

Static Imaging

Static imaging demonstrated a hot spot in the axilla which represented the sentinel node. The overlying skin was marked with an indelible pen.

Operative Findings

The patient underwent a modified radical mastectomy and sentinel node biopsy. Patent blue dye was injected prior to incision. A single hot node was identified with the Neoprobe 1500. This node had taken up blue dye as well.

Histology

Histology confirmed the diagnosis of grade 1 invasive lobular carcinoma. The tumour was 3.5 cm in its maximum dimension. The sentinel node was not involved with metastatic carcinoma on H & E staining or immunohistochemistry. None of the remaining 15 axillary lymph nodes were involved. Oestrogen receptor status was positive.

Teaching Point

This case demonstrates that subdermal injection of ^{99m}Tc-colloid with average particle size of less than 400 nm leads to a very rapid progression of tracer on dynamic imaging in central breast carcinoma owing to a rich subareolar lymphatic plexus.

Static Imaging

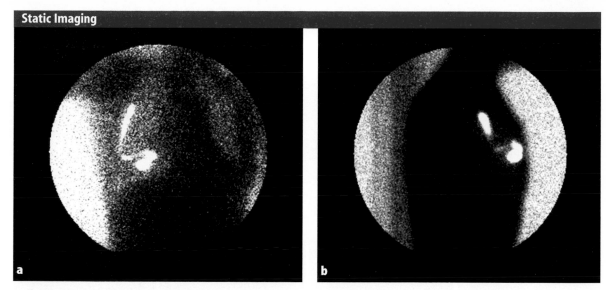

a Anterior-oblique view
b Lateral view

Histology

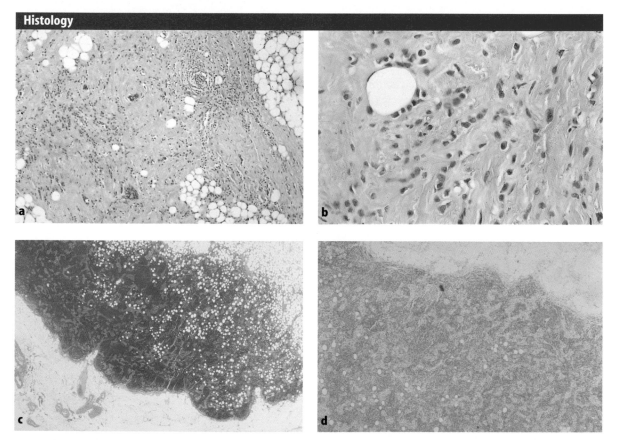

a Grade-1 invasive lobular carcinoma (H & E)
b Magnified view showing indian file pattern and intracytoplasmic lumina (H & E)
c Sentinel node partially replaced by fat. No evidence of malignancy (H & E)
d Negative sentinel node (MNF 116)

Upper Outer Quadrant Breast Carcinoma

A 60-year-old female presented with a 2-cm lump in the upper outer quadrant of the right breast which had been noted 6 weeks previously. There were no palpable axillary lymph nodes.

Mammography, ultrasound and fine-needle aspiration cytology confirmed the clinical impression of breast cancer.

Operative Findings

The sentinel node was easily identified using the Neoprobe 1500 gamma detection probe with a collimator attached to the probe to prevent scatter.

Dynamic Imaging

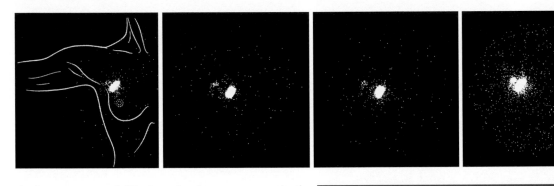

As there was no visible lymphatic tract or sentinel node on the early dynamic data acquisition and it was felt that this might be due to the close proximity of the injection site of the tracer in respect to the axilla, further imaging was carried out. On retracting the breast downward and medially, the sentinel node became apparent (see also Chap. 6, Fig. 2).

Static Imaging

The static acquisition confirmed the site of the sentinel node, and the lateral view was very helpful in delineating the sentinel node and giving information on its depth.

Histology

Histology revealed grade 2 invasive ductal carcinoma. The sentinel node was not involved on H & E staining and this was confirmed by immunohistochemistry. None of the other lymph nodes obtained from axillary node clearance contained tumour.

Teaching Point

In upper outer quadrant lesions, it is best to retract the breast downward and medially so that the injection site does not overshadow the site of the sentinel node. Lateral view acquisition is very helpful in these cases. The gamma detection probe is best used with a collimator to avoid scatter radiation from the injection site.

Static Imaging

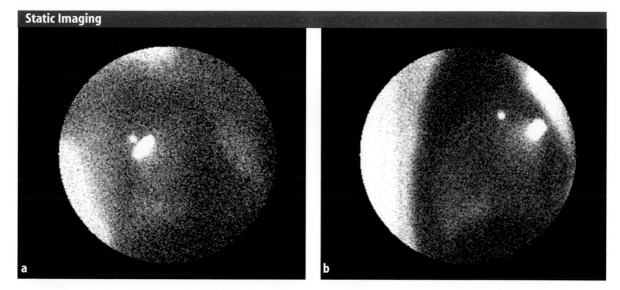

a Anterior-oblique view
b Lateral view

Histology

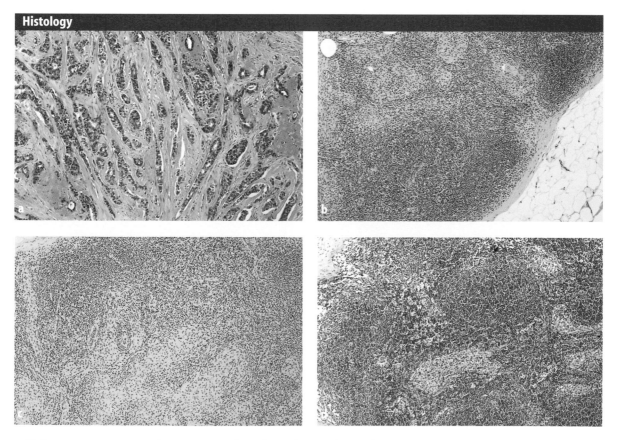

a Primary tumour – grade 2 invasive ductal carcinoma (H & E)
b Negative sentinel node (H & E)
c Negative sentinel node (MNF 116)
d Non-sentinel node not involved (H & E)

Upper Inner Quadrant Breast Carcinoma

A 50-year-old female presented with a lump in her left breast. On examination there was a 2-cm ill-defined mass in the upper inner quadrant of the left breast. There was no evidence of axillary lymphadenopathy. Investigations confirmed the diagnosis of breast cancer.

Lymphoscintigraphy

Lymphoscintigraphy was performed after injection of 15MBq of ^{99m}Tc-colloidal albumin. During injection it was felt that it was administered deeper than usual in the subcutaneous fat. Dynamic acquisition and static acquisition did not reveal any sentinel lymph node. Delayed imaging 18 h after injection also failed to show focal uptake. As the patient's operation had to be postponed, she underwent repeat imaging 2 days later.

Dynamic Imaging

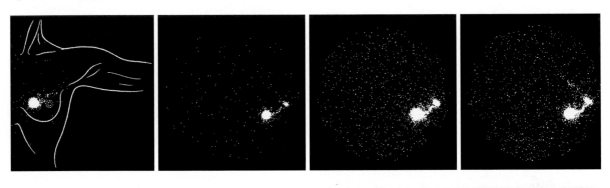

Repeat dynamic imaging revealed a rapid transit of tracer through the lymphatic channels to the first drainage basin, with visualisation of the sentinel node.

Static imaging confirmed the presence of at least two areas of focal activity which were considered to be the sentinel nodes.

Operative Findings

At operation 2 ml of patent blue dye was injected at the tumour site. On exploration of the axilla with the Neoprobe 1500, a hot node was found at level 1. After excising the node, gamma detection probe was re-applied and this revealed another lymph node proximal to the first one; this second node showed more radioactivity and had taken up the blue dye as well. This was also biopsied and the patient underwent wide local excision and axillary node clearance.

Histology

Histology revealed a 2.5-cm, grade 3 invasive ductal carcinoma with vascular permeation. Two sentinel nodes were replaced with metastatic tumour. An additional three lymph nodes from axillary clearance contained metastases.

Teaching Point

This case demonstrates that the injection technique is an important variable in sentinel node localisation. It was felt that the first injection was delivered into the subcutaneous tissue and the tracer did not move due to the poor lymphatic supply in this layer. Subsequent injection into the subdermal lymphatic plexus was successful in demonstrating the sentinel nodes.

Static Imaging

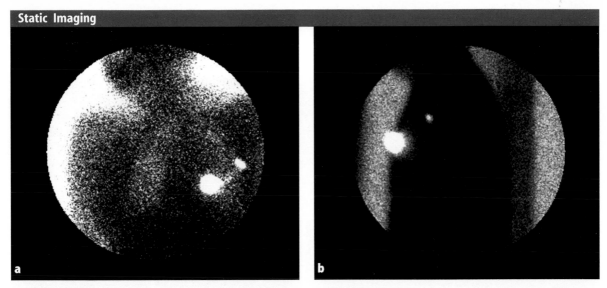

a Anterior-oblique view
b Lateral view

Histology

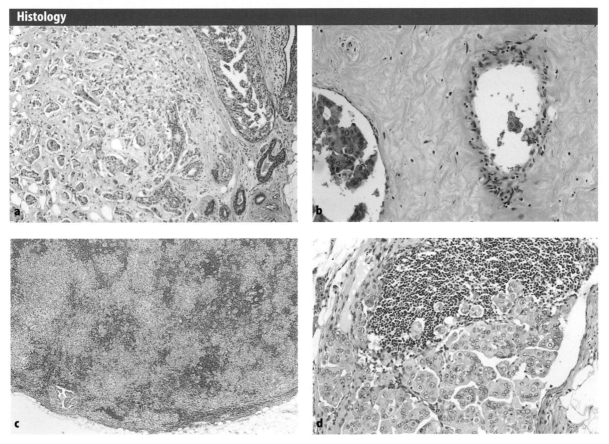

a Grade-3 invasive ductal carcinoma (H & E)
b High power view showing vascular invasion (H & E)
c The sentinel node is extensively replaced with metastatic carcinoma (H & E)
d High power view of the SLN, replaced with metastatic carcinoma (H & E)

Internal Mammary Sentinel Node in Upper Outer Quadrant Breast Carcinoma

A 47-year-old female presented with a lump in her right breast. On examination, she had an ill-defined 4 cm lump in the upper outer quadrant of the right breast and there was a palpable axillary lymph node. Investigations confirmed the diagnosis of breast cancer.

Dynamic Imaging

Operative Findings

At operation, there was gross evidence of disease in the axilla with nodal involvement. There was no area of focal uptake on applying the Neoprobe 1500 in the axilla. The patient underwent qua-

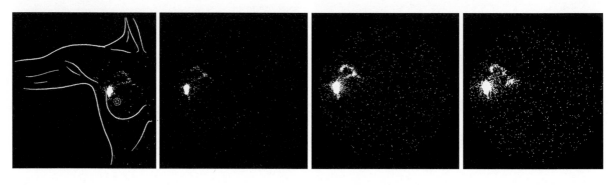

Dynamic imaging showed surprisingly, progression of the tracer medially towards the internal mammary chain. There was an area of focal uptake which was thought to be an internal mammary node.

Static Imaging

Static imaging failed to show any uptake at the axilla and confirmed the presence of an internal mammary lymph node.

drantectomy and complete axillary node clearance. It is not the policy of our surgical unit to biopsy internal mammary lymph nodes.

Histology

Histology revealed a grade 3 invasive ductal carcinoma with intravascular invasion. Oestrogen receptor was 60% positive. Six axillary lymph nodes were involved with metastatic carcinoma, two of which were completely replaced with tumour. There was also evidence of extranodal spread of cancer into axillary fat.

Teaching Points

Patients with clinically involved axillary lymph nodes should not be considered for sentinel node biopsy. In this case, uptake in the internal mammary chain was thought to be due to a diversion of lymph flow, as a result of a complete replacement of a number of axillary lymph nodes with metastatic cancer. Demonstration of internal mammary nodes is, in our experience, rare. Nevertheless, it represents a special case. There is controversy as to the significance of the sentinel node method in these cases.

Static Imaging

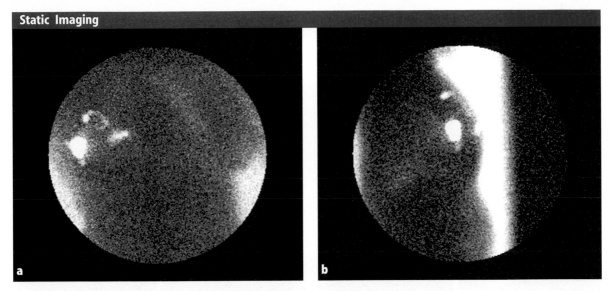

a Anterior-oblique view showing uptake in internal mammary node
b Lateral view

Histology

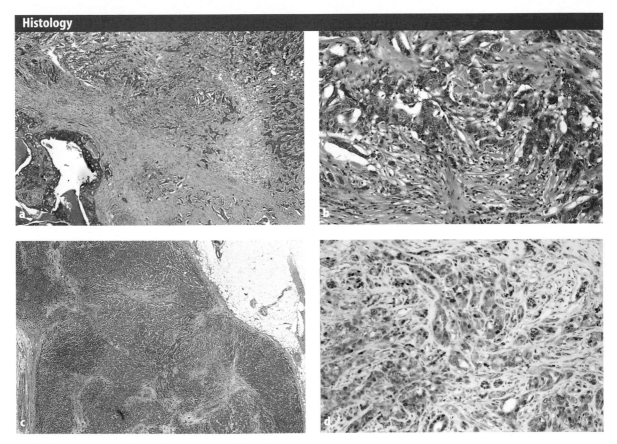

a Grade-3 invasive ductal carcinoma (H & E)
b Higher magnification of the tumour (H & E)
c Axillary lymph node completely replaced with metastatic carcinoma (H & E)
d Oestrogen receptor positive (ER Positive)

Micrometastases in Sentinel Nodes

A 42-year-old female presented with a small lump in the right breast. On examination she had a 1 cm lump in the upper outer quadrant and there was no evidence of axillary lymphadenopathy. Investigations confirmed the diagnosis of invasive breast carcinoma. She consented for wide local excision of the primary tumour and sentinel node biopsy only.

Histology

Histology revealed a grade 3 invasive medullary carcinoma of the breast. Two sentinel nodes were not involved on H & E staining but on immunohistochemical (IHC) staining for pancytokeratin marker (MNF 116), both nodes showed evidence of micrometastasis.

Dynamic Imaging

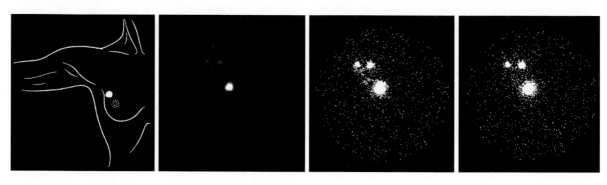

Dynamic imaging revealed a lymphatic tract in the direction of the axilla which branched before reaching the lymph node. Two areas of increased focal uptake gradually became evident.

Static Imaging

Static imaging confirmed the presence of two sentinel nodes on the anterior oblique view. The lateral view revealed that one node was proximal to the other.

Operative Findings

On exploring the axilla, a small sentinel node was found using the Neoprobe 1500. The node was at level 1 but adhered to the chest wall. The second sentinel node was at level 2 and both nodes were blue.

Teaching Point

This case clearly demonstrates the advantage of sentinel node biopsy. It led to a more sensitive IHC examination which made it possible to detect the micrometastasis and accurately stage the patient. This had a significant bearing on the decision making regarding adjuvant therapy.

Static Imaging

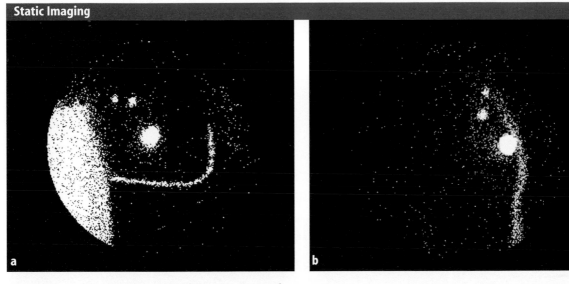

a Anterior-oblique view with a line source marker
b Lateral view with a line source marker

Histology

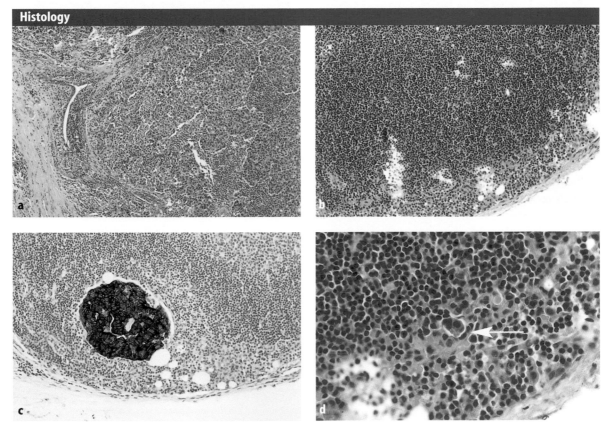

a Grade-3 medullary carcinoma (H & E)
b The sentinel node was negative on H & E staining
c The sentinel node shows evidence of metastasis on immunohistochemistry (MNF 116)
d Review of H & E staining confirms metastatic deposits (*arrow*)

Fat Replacement of Sentinel Node

A 70-year-old female presented with a lump in the right breast. On examination, there was a 1.5-cm soft mass in the upper inner quadrant with no clinical evidence of axillary node involvement. Investigations confirmed the diagnosis of breast carcinoma.

to be difficult. A weakly radioactive node was detected with the Neoprobe 1500. The nodal activity was only 3 times the background activity and the sentinel node had partly taken up the blue dye.

Dynamic Imaging

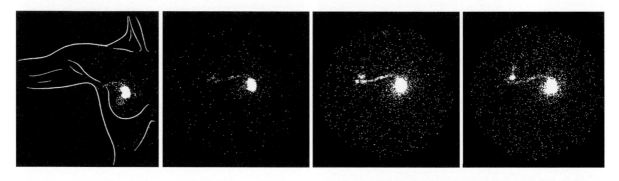

Dynamic imaging revealed a lymphatic tract running towards the axilla within 5 min of injection of radiotracer.

Static Imaging

Static imaging confirmed a single area of increased focal activity in the axilla. There was no uptake in the internal mammary chain.

Operative Findings

Two millilitres of patent blue dye was injected subdermally at the tumour site. On exploration of the axilla, sentinel node localisation proved

Histology

It was very difficult to prepare the frozen section slides. On H & E staining paraffin sections revealed that the sentinel node was almost completely replaced with fat. The sentinel node did not show any evidence of metastatic carcinoma on H & E staining or immunohistochemistry. None of the nodes from axillary clearance were involved with carcinoma. The primary tumour was confirmed as a grade 1 invasive ductal carcinoma.

Teaching point

Fat replacement of lymph nodes in elderly patients is a recognised entity. If the sentinel node is replaced with fat, its localization is difficult due to decreased capacity of the node to retain the tracer. This can also make frozen sections difficult to prepare and interpret. Increasing the dosage of radiopharmaceutical may help to overcome this problem in elderly patients.

Static Imaging

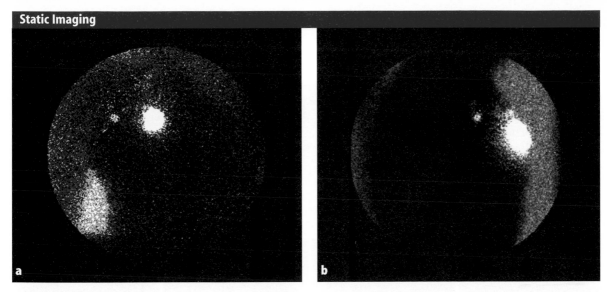

a Anterior-oblique view
b Lateral view

Histology

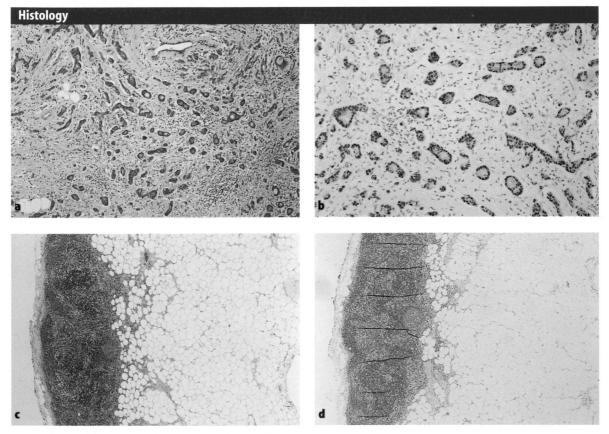

a Grade-1 invasive ductal carcinoma (H & E)
b Oestrogen receptor positive (ER Positive)
c The sentinel node replaced with fat with only a thin rim of residual lymphoid tissue
d Negative sentinel node (MNF 116)

Reduced Functional Capacity of Lymph Node

A 62-year-old female presented with a dimple in the lower outer quadrant of the left breast. On examination, there was a 1.7-cm hard lump underlying the deformed area. There was no clinical evidence of axillary lymph node involvement. The diagnosis of breast carcinoma was confirmed on triple assessment.

was biopsied and in order to check the residual activity the probe was re-applied in the wound and a node with much weaker activity was identified distally with activity twice the background. This was also biopsied and sent separately for histology. The patient underwent quadrantectomy and axillary lymph node dissection.

Dynamic Imaging

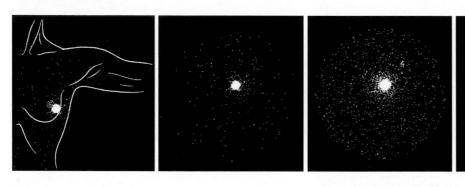

There was relatively slow uptake of the radiopharmaceutical and no obvious tract was visible. The area of increased focal uptake was evident within 25 min of injection.

Static Imaging

Static imaging confirmed on area of increased focal activity in the axilla. The overlying skin was marked.

Histology

Histology revealed a grade 3 invasive ductal carcinoma with evidence of ductal carcinoma in situ. The sentinel node showed heavy infiltration with metastatic carcinoma, but the lower node with much less tracer activity revealed even more extensive infiltration with metastatic cancer. Oestrogen receptor status was negative.

Operative Findings

There was macroscopic evidence of axillary involvement. A very hot sentinel node was identified with the Neoprobe 1500, higher up at level 1. This

Teaching Point

This case demonstrates the reduced functional capacity of a lymph node because of extensive infiltration with metastatic carcinoma, lead to minimal uptake of the radiopharmaceutical. This phenomenon is a potential pitfall in sentinel node biopsy.

Static Imaging

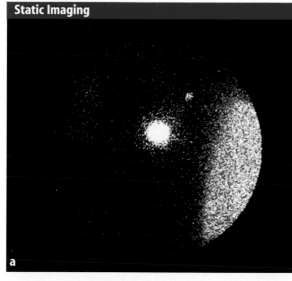
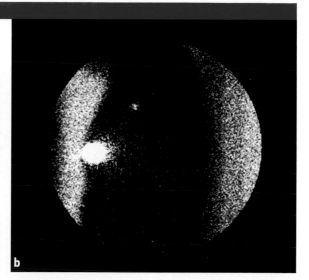

a Left anterior-oblique view   **b** Lateral view

Histology

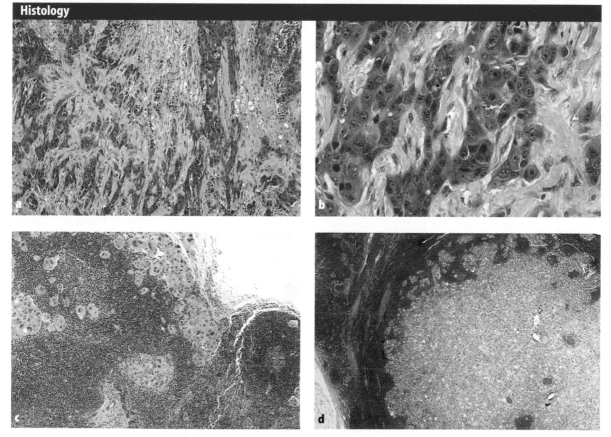

a Low power view of invasive ductal carcinoma grade-3 (H & E)
b High power view of invasive ductal carcinoma grade-3 (H & E)
c "Hot" sentinel node with foci of metastatic carcinoma (H & E)
d Lower node with less tracer activity showing almost complete effacement by metastatic carcinoma (H & E)

"Langer's Axillary Arch" and the Sentinel Node

A 43-year-old female presented with a 5-month history of a lump in the right breast. On examination there was an ill-defined lump in the upper inner quadrant of the right breast. There were no palpable axillary lymph nodes. Triple assessment confirmed the diagnosis of breast carcinoma.

primary site and on exploring the axilla, a blue and hot sentinel node was found superficially, just underneath the axillary fat, and was biopsied. During axillary node dissection it was evident that the sentinel node was overlying the Langer's axillary arch, which is a relatively rare anatomical

Dynamic Imaging

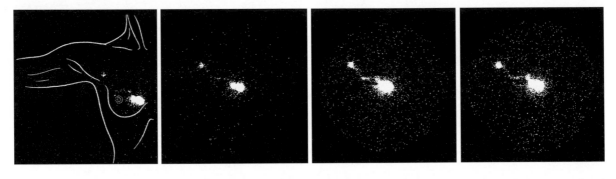

There was rapid transit of the radiopharmaceutical towards the axilla and an increased area of focal accumulation of radioactivity was evident within 5 min. There was no evidence of internal mammary nodal uptake.

variation of the insertion of the latissimus dorsi muscle. An anomalous (axillopectoral) muscle extends from the lateral border of the latissimus dorsi to the humeral insertion of the pectoralis major.

Static Imaging

On the anterior-oblique view, there was focal uptake of radioactivity high in the axilla, and this was confirmed on the lateral view.

Operating Findings

It was easy to localise the sentinel node with the Neoprobe 1500, before the incision was made. 1.5 ml of patent blue dye was injected at the

Histology

Histology revealed a 1 cm, grade 1 invasive ductal carcinoma. The sentinel node was free of metastatic tumour and none of the other axillary lymph nodes were involved with metastatic cancer. Immunohistochemical staining (MNF 116) was negative for micrometastasis.

Teaching Point

This case demonstrates a rare anatomical variation encountered during sentinel node biopsy. It is responsible for an unusually superficial plane of the sentinel node. This was easily detected with the Neoprobe 1500. Anatomical anaomalies should be kept in mind during the sentinel node biopsy procedure.

Static Imaging

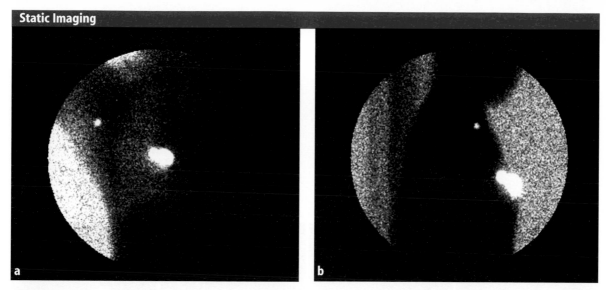

a Right anterior-oblique view
b Lateral view

Histology

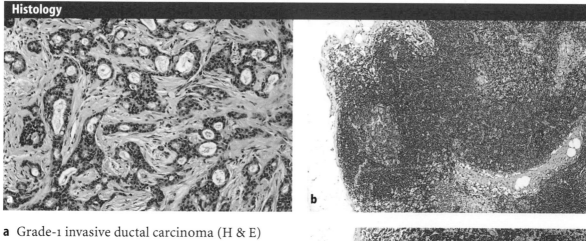

a Grade-1 invasive ductal carcinoma (H & E)
b Negative sentinel node (H & E)

c Negative non-sentinel node (H & E)

Presence of Blue Dye in Macrophages

A 70-year-female presented with a lump in the upper pole of the breast above the nipple. On examination, there was a 2.5-cm ill-defined lump with no clinical evidence of axillary involvement. The diagnosis of carcinoma was confirmed on triple assessment.

Dynamic Imaging

Operative Findings

With the help of the Neoprobe 1500 it was possible to locate the sentinel nodes. These were located posteriorly along the medial pectoral group, in close proximity to the chest wall. Both nodes had also taken up the patent blue dye.

There was relatively slow uptake of colloidal particles on dynamic imaging with no lymphatic tract visible. Two areas of increased focal uptake became evident in the axilla.

Static Imaging

Static imaging confirmed the presence of two areas of increased focal accumulation of the radiotracer. The overlying skin was marked.

Imprint Cytology and Histology

There was no evidence of malignancy on imprint cytology. Interestingly, presence of the patent blue dye in a macrophage was noted on imprint cytology. Histology of the sentinel node did not reveal any evidence of metastatic deposits on H & E staining or immunohistochemistry (MNF 116).

Teaching Point

This case demonstrates that gamma probe-guided surgery is very helpful in guiding the surgeon towards sentinel nodes in a less easily accessible location. The finding of blue dye in a macrophage on imprint cytology represents a good demonstration of nodal uptake of particles by phagocytosis.

Static Imaging

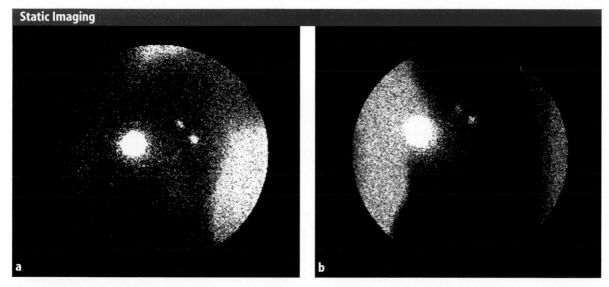

a Left anterior-oblique view
b Lateral view

Histology

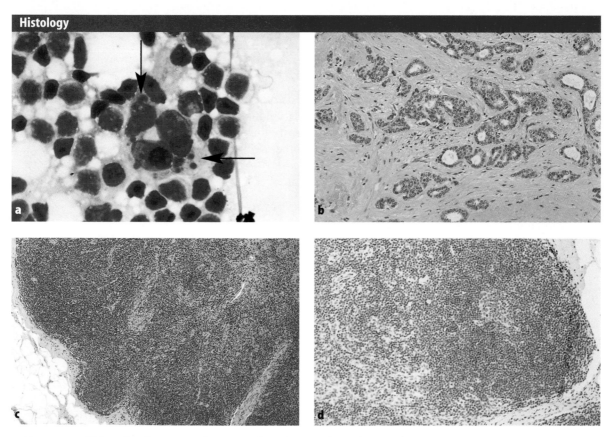

a Presence of blue dye in macrophages on imprint cytology (*arrows*)
b Grade-1 invasive ductal carcinoma (H & E)
c Negative sentinel node (H & E)
d Negative sentinel node (MNF 116)

Subdermal Injection of Radiocolloid and Peritumoral Injection of the Blue Dye

A 73-year-old female presented with a dimple in the right breast. On examination there was an ill-defined lump underlying the deformity. There was no clinical evidence of axillary lymph node involvement. The diagnosis of invasive breast carcinoma was confirmed on triple assessment.

The site of the sentinel node was verified with the Neoprobe 1500. After waiting for 5 min, the axilla was explored. The hot sentinel node was identified with the probe. The sentinel node had taken up the blue dye.

Dynamic Imaging

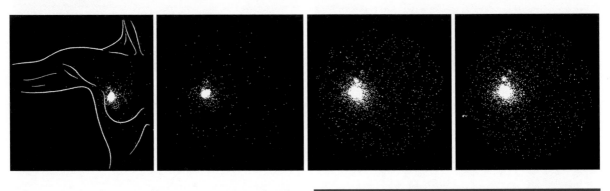

Fifteen MBq of ^{99m}Tc-Albures was injected sub-dermally. There was no evidence of a lymphatic tract on initial acquisition. As the site of injection was close to the axilla, by retracting the breast medially and downward, an area of increased focal activity became evident.

Static Imaging

This confirmed the presence of increased focal activity and in particular the lateral view was very helpful in giving the depth perception.

Operative Findings

Two millilitres of patent blue dye was injected into the breast parenchyma in a peritumoral fashion.

Histology

Histology revealed a 1.7-cm, grade 2 invasive ductal carcinoma. The sentinel node was not involved with the metastatic carcinoma and none of 18 other axillary nodes were involved.

Teaching Point

This case validates the hypothesis that the dermal and parenchymal lymphatics of the breast communicate and follow a common pathway to the axillary lymph nodes. This case also demonstrates that in upper outer carcinoma of breast, downward and medial retraction of the breast is helpful in delineating the sentinel node.

Static Imaging

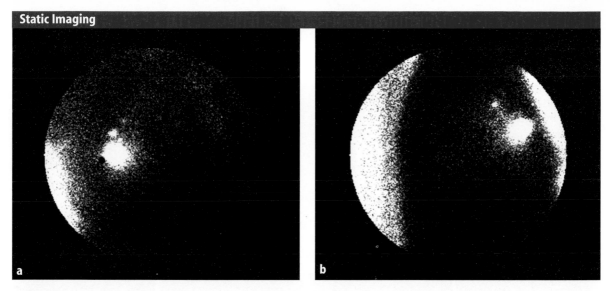

a Right anterior-oblique view
b Lateral view

Histology

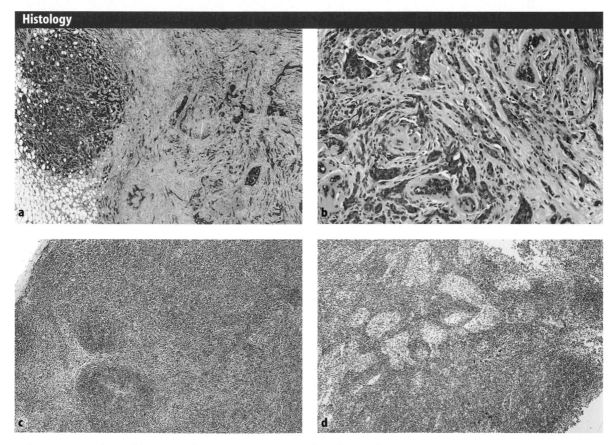

a Low power view of invasive ductal carcinoma grade-2 (H & E)
b High power view of invasive ductal carcinoma grade-2 (H & E)
c Negative sentinel node (H & E)
d Negative sentinel node (MNF 116). A few positively stained cells are seen but these are macrophages

Male Breast Carcinoma

A 60-year-old male presented with a 2-month history of inverted left nipple with an underlying lump. The patient was on warfarin sodium, anti-coagulant therapy and low-dose aspirin for aortic valve replacement. On examination he was grossly obese with an inverted left nipple and a 2 cm subareolar lump, but there were no palpable axillary nodes. Standard investigations confirmed the diagnosis of breast cancer.

Operative Findings

At the primary tumour site, 1.5 ml patent blue dye was injected. On exploring the axilla, using the Neoprobe 1500 gamma detection probe, a hot but not blue node was identified at level 1. Higher up, a blue node was found which was not hot. The patient underwent mastectomy and axillary clearance.

Dynamic Imaging

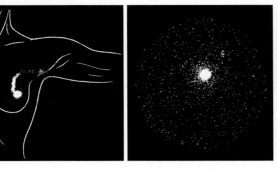 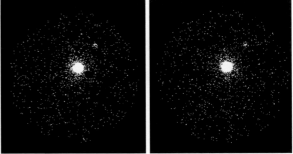

The lymphatic tract became evident immediately, with rapid movement of colloidal particles towards the axilla.

Imprint Cytology and Histology

Imprint cytology confirmed that the hot node was involved with metastatic cancer cells and the blue node was free of tumour (see Chap. 10, Figs. 6 and 7). Histology revealed a 2-cm, grade 3 invasive ductal carcinoma with no vascular invasion. Histological examination of the sentinel node confirmed the cytology findings. The sentinel node was the only lymph node involved and all other 11 axillary nodes were free of tumour.

Static Imaging

Static imaging confirmed the presence of a sentinel node in the axilla and the overlying skin was marked with an indelible pen.

Teaching Point

Sentinel node biopsy should be considered in high-risk patients who are on anticoagulant therapy to reduce postoperative morbidity. Imprint cytology was valuable in this case and correctly predicted the sentinel node status.

Static Imaging

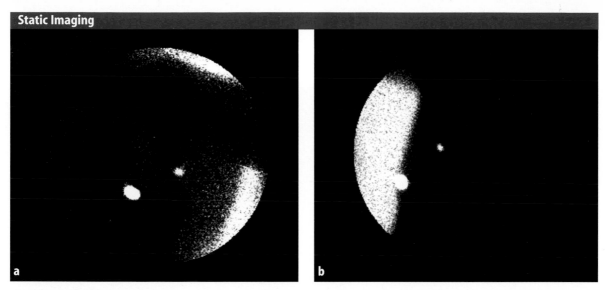

a Left anterior-oblique view
b Lateral view

Histology

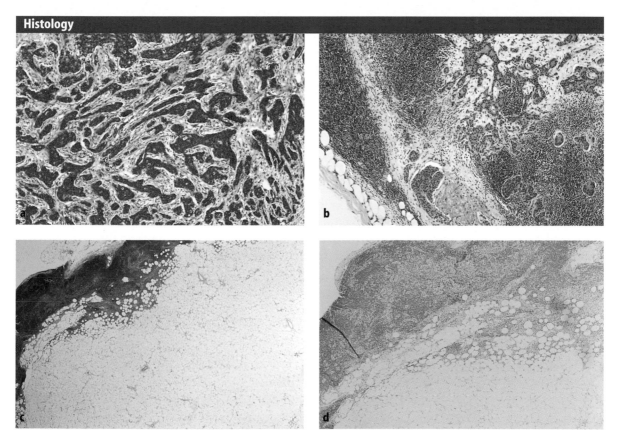

a Grade-3 invasive ductal carcinoma (H & E)
b The hot sentinel node involved with metastatic deposits (H & E)
c The blue and cold node almost completely replaced with fat and not involved with carcinoma (H & E)
d Negative immunohistochemistry (MNF 116)

Malignant Melanoma of the Calf

A 51-year-old woman presented with a mole on her left calf. Excision biopsy confirmed the diagnosis of malignant melanoma, with a Breslow thickness of 6.8 mm and Clark's level 5. She subsequently had a wider excision which did not show any evidence of residual tumour. On examination, the scar of the previous excision was obvious with no palpable inguinal lymph nodes. The patient underwent lymphatic scintigraphy and sentinel node biopsy.

Operative Findings

Through a 2-cm incision, a sentinel node was easily detected using the gamma detection probe and Patent Blue dye.

Dynamic Imaging

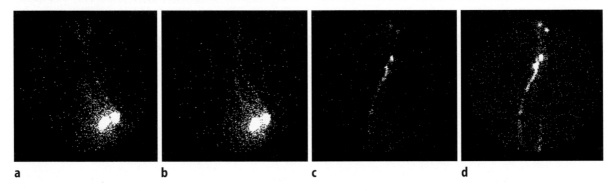

a   b   c   d

a, b Dynamic imaging at the injection site (leg)

c, d Dynamic imaging at the groin and pelvis

On dynamic imaging of the injection site it was apparent that the drainage was towards the groin region. Further acquisition was obtained from the groin and pelvic region and the sentinel node could be identified.

Histology

Histology revealed that the sentinel node was free of tumour on H & E staining and this was confirmed on immunohistochemistry.

Static Imaging

Multiple lymph nodes were seen. The first node that became obvious in the groin on dynamic acquisition was regarded as a sentinel node and the overlying skin was marked.

Teaching Point

Dynamic imaging is very important in lymphatic mapping in malignant melanoma. It helps to determine the direction of drainage to the lymphatic basin and also visualises the first lymph node.

Static imaging

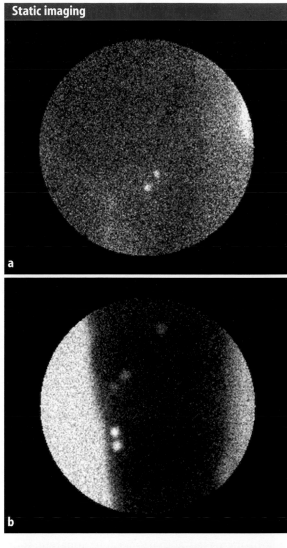

Anterior view **a**
Lateral view **b**

Histology

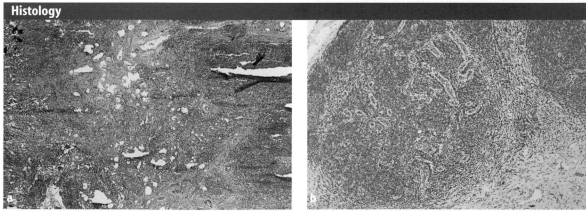

a Negative sentinel node (frozen section)
b Negative sentinel node (HMB-45)

Malignant Melanoma of the Thigh

A 40-year-old female presented with a long-standing mole on the lateral aspect of the right thigh which had started to bleed and to grow. She had no palpable lymph nodes in the groin. Excision biopsy of the mole confirmed the diagnosis of malignant melanoma, Breslow thickness 1.3 mm, Clark's level 4. Staging investigations including CT scan of abdomen and thorax were normal.

Lymphoscintigraphy
Lymphoscintigraphy was performed by injecting 7 MBq ^{99m}Tc-albumin colloid at four sites along the excision biopsy scar.

Dynamic Imaging

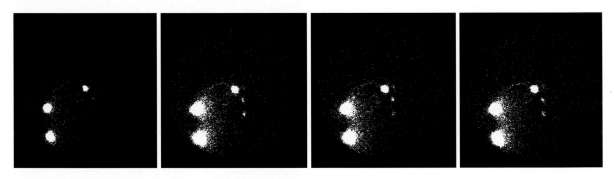

Dynamic imaging confirmed rapid transit of the isotopes towards the right inguinal region. A focal area of increased activity became apparent soon after injection.

Static Imaging

On the anterior view, the sentinel node was clearly evident. On the lateral view, the injection sites were clearly seen and a sentinel node was apparent. There was also a focal area of activity posteriorly which did not correspond to any lymphatic basin. This was due to contamination of the patient's dress during injection.

Operative Findings
As the sentinel node was close to the injection site, the Neoprobe 1500 was used with a collimator. A blue and hot node was biopsied through a 2.5-cm groin incision. The patient also had a wider excision of the primary site.

Histology

There was no evidence of metastatic deposits in the sentinel node on H & E staining and immunohistochemistry. The wider excision did not show any evidence of residual tumour.

Teaching Point

Care needs to be taken that there is no contamination during injection of the radiopharmaceutical as the artefact can mimic a sentinel node.

Static Imaging

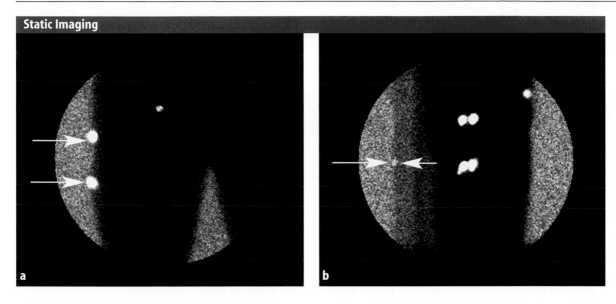

a Anterior view (*arrows* show injection site)
b Lateral view (*arrows* contamination)

Histology

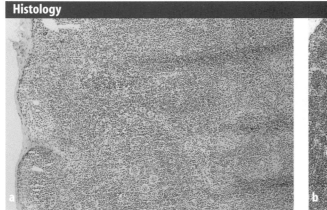

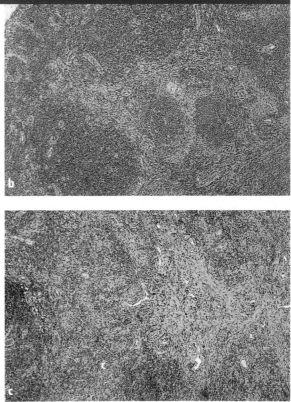

a Frozen section shows no evidence of metastatic deposit in the sentinel node
b H & E staining shows no evidence of metastatic deposits

c Negative immunohistochemistry (S-100)

Malignant Melanoma with Previous Excision

A 46-year-old man who underwent wide excision and skin grafting of malignant melanoma of the left calf was referred for sentinel node biopsy. Histology revealed Clark's level 4 and a Breslow thickness of 4 mm. There were no palpable inguinal lymph nodes. Screening investigations, including CT and MRI scans, showed no evidence of distant metastases.

Lymphoscintigraphy

As there was a large circular area in the calf with a partly taken split thickness skin graft, 4 MBq of ^{99m}Tc-albumin colloid was injected at each of four sites around the previous excision cavity, at the 3, 6, 9 and 12 o'clock positions.

Dynamic Imaging

Static imaging revealed a sentinel node in the left groin and the overlying skin was marked with a indelible pen.

Operative Findings

At operation 0.5 ml of patent blue dye was injected at the four sites mentioned earlier. The groin was explored through a 2.5-cm incision. A hot node was identified with the Neoprobe 1500. It was blue and it was biopsied.

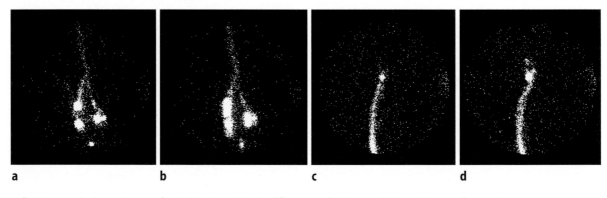

a   b   c   d

a, b Dynamic imaging at the injection site (calf)   **c, d** Dynamic imaging at the groin

Dynamic imaging demonstrated rapid progression of the radioactive tracer towards the left groin. The lymphatic tracts from the injection sites joined into a common lymphatic trunk. Dynamic acquisition of the thigh and groin confirmed a single trunk leading to a sentinel node.

Teaching point

Imprint Cytology and Histology

Imprint cytology did not show any evidence of metastasis in the sentinel node. Histological analysis on frozen sections, H & E sections and immunohistochemical examination did not reveal any nodal involvement.

Sentinel node biopsy is feasible in malignant melanoma with previous wide excision and skin grafting. Dynamic acquisition is a mandatory part of imaging. Imprint cytology findings corresponded to H & E and immunohistochemistry.

Static Imaging

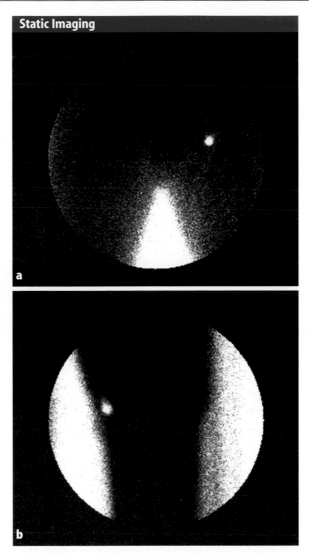

Anterior view **a**
Lateral view **b**

Histology

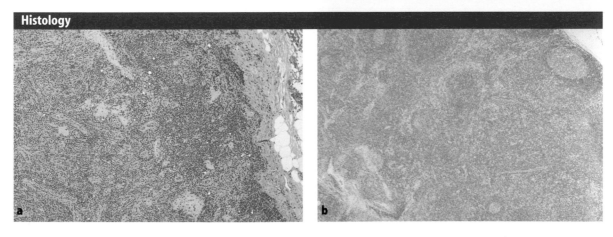

a Negative sentinel node (H & E)
b Negative sentinel node (HMB-45)

Malignant Melanoma of the Upper Arm

An 80-year-old female presented with a mole on her left upper arm. There was no evidence of axillary lymphadenopathy. Excision biopsy confirmed the diagnosis of malignant melanoma, with a Breslow thickness of 7.5 mm and Clark's level 4. There was no evidence of distant metastasis. She underwent sentinel node biopsy and wider excision at the site of the primary lesion.

Operative Findings

Patent blue dye was injected at four sites around the previous excision biopsy scar. A small incision was made over the site of maximum counts determined by the Neoprobe 1500. Two sentinel nodes were easily detected with the probe and they had taken up the blue dye as well.

Dynamic Imaging

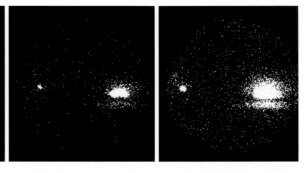

On dynamic imaging, there was rapid transit of the tracer towards the axilla, with an area of increased focal activity evident within 5 min after the injection.

Static Imaging

Static imaging revealed one node in the axilla, regarded as the sentinel node. The overlying skin was marked.

Imprint Cytology and Histology

Imprint cytology confirmed evidence of metastatic deposits in the sentinel nodes. Histological analysis of the nodes confirmed their replacement with metastatic melanoma on H & E staining and immunohistochemical staining (HMB-45, S100).

Teaching Point

The sentinel node technique was helpful in proper staging of this elderly patient without any morbidity. Care must be taken to survey the lymphatic basin for residual a radioactivity. This case also demonstrates a good correlation between imprint cytology and definitive histology of the sentinel node.

Static Imaging

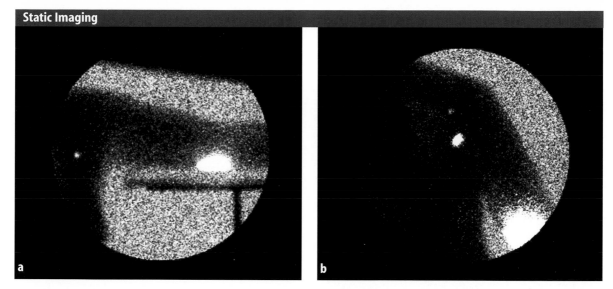

a Left anterior-oblique view
b Left anterior view

Histology

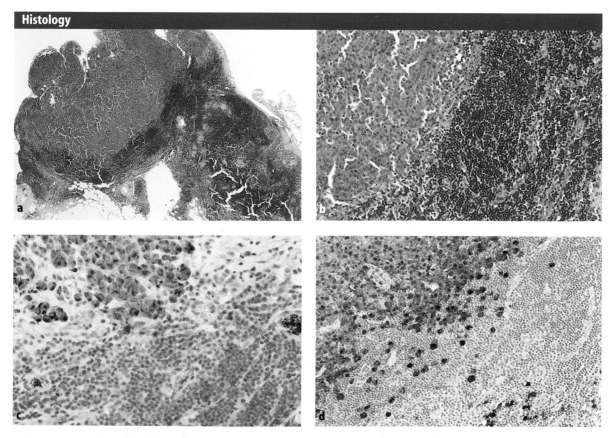

a Low power view showing effacement of sentinel node by metastatic melanoma (H & E)
b High power view of metastatic melanoma in sentinel node (H & E)
c Metastatic melanoma (HMB-45)
d Metastatic melanoma (S100)

Colon Carcinoma

A 57-year-old Cantonese lady presented with a history of rectal bleeding and abdominal pain.

Investigations
Colonoscopy revealed a constricting lesion in the sigmoid colon which was biopsied. This confirmed the diagnosis of sigmoid carcinoma.

Operative Findings
A stenosing carcinoma of the sigmoid colon was evident. 2 ml of patent blue dye was injected sub-serosally on either side of the tumour. The sigmoid and the descending colon were mobilised. A few grossly abnormal lymph nodes were noted in the mesocolon. A blue node became apparent distal to these pathological nodes which looked grossly normal. It was obvious that the dye had bypassed the involved lymph nodes.

Histology
Histology revealed an invasive, moderately differentiated, Dukes' stage C adenocarcinoma at the primary site. The sentinel node was free of the tumour and the two lymph nodes that looked abnormal were completely replaced by metastatic tumour. Immunohistochemistry of the sentinel node was also negative.

Teaching Point

This case demonstrates a skip phenomenon. This is due to complete replacement of the lymph node with carcinoma, which leads to directional flow changes in lymphatic channels and consequently a false-negative result. In colon cancers, sentinel node detection with blue dye is very useful. Progress is being made with the radionuclide detection of the sentinel node.

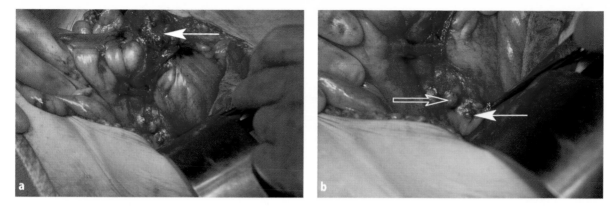

a Subserosal injection of patent blue dye around sigmoid carcinoma (*arrow*)
b Grossly involved lymph node is not stained with blue dye (*empty arrow*); distal normal lymph node has taken up blue dye (*solid arrow*)

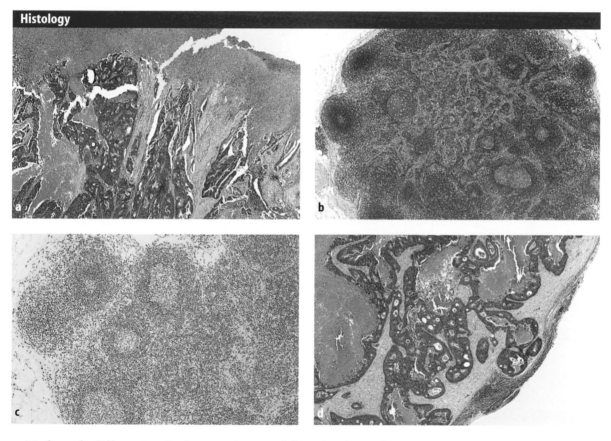

Histology

a Moderately differentiated adenocarcinoma of the colon (H & E)
b Negative sentinel node (H & E)
c Negative sentinel node (MNF 116)
d Non-sentinel node in the mesocolon is heavily infiltrated with metastatic adenocarcinoma (H & E)

Rectal Carcinoma

An 88-year-old female presented with changed bowel habits and passing blood per rectum. On digital rectal examination, there was a stenosing lesion, 6 cm from the anal verge. Biopsy of this lesion confirmed the diagnosis of rectal carcinoma. Barium enema also confirmed the findings and did not show any other colonic lesions. The patient underwent a low anterior resection with total mesorectal excision and sentinel node biopsy using patent blue dye.

Injection Technique

A proctoscope was inserted into the rectum whilst the patient was under general anaesthesia. 2 ml of patent blue dye was injected submucosally at the level of the tumour (see Chap. 5, Fig. 11).

Operative Findings

The left colon and rectum were fully mobilised and low anterior resection with complete meso-rectal excision was performed. On examination of mesorectal tissues, most of the lymph nodes had taken up the blue dye and the blue node closest to the lesion was investigated separately as a sentinel node.

Histology

Histology revealed Dukes' stage B adenocarcinoma. The sentinel node was free of tumour on H & E staining and immunohistochemistry. All other mesorectal lymph nodes were free of tumour.

Teaching point

Sentinel node biopsy for rectal carcinoma using patent blue dye is technically difficult owing to the rapid progression of the patent blue dye from one node to another. This problem can be overcome by using a radioisotope technique. In this case, the sentinel node correctly predicted the status of other nodes in the lymphatic basin.

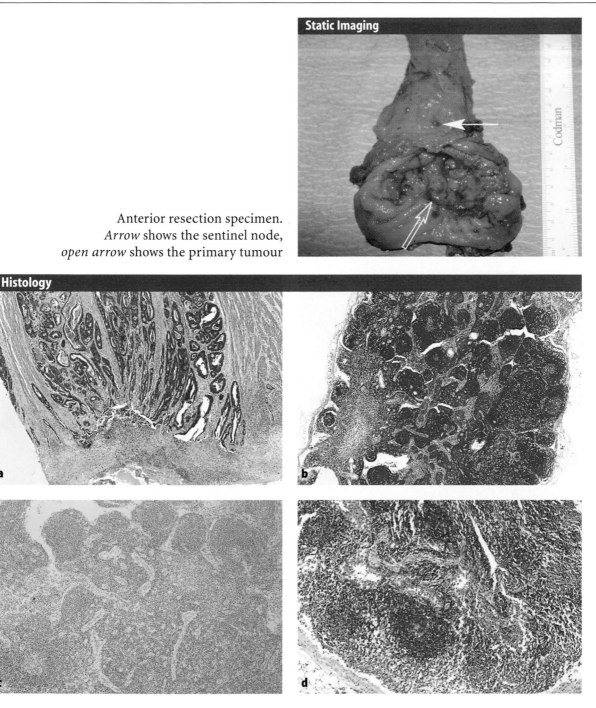

Anterior resection specimen.
Arrow shows the sentinel node,
open arrow shows the primary tumour

Static Imaging

Histology

a Moderately differentiated adenocarcinoma of the rectum (H & E)
b The sentinel node showing reactive changes (H & E)
c Negative sentinel node (MNF 116)
d Negative non-sentinel, mesorectal node (H & E)

Penile Carcinoma

A 42-year-old male was referred for sentinel node biopsy of the left groin. Four years previously he had, been diagnosed as having a squamous cell carcinoma of the penis, which was treated with circumcision and cauterisation. He developed metastases to the right groin after 3 years; these were excised. A year after this, he underwent radical groin dissection for recurrence in the groin. He subsequently developed lymphoedema of the right lower limb.

Lymphoscintigraphy

After application of local anaesthetic cream on the dorsum of the penis just proximal to the site of cauterisation, 15 MBq of ^{99m}Tc-Albures was injected subdermally (see Chap. 5, Fig. 12).

Dynamic Imaging

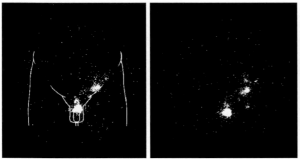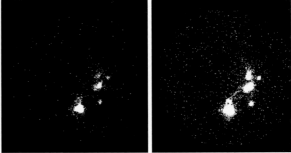

Dynamic imaging revealed that there was rapid movement of colloidal particles towards the left groin. The lymphatic tract was well demonstrated. Focal uptake of tracer was evident in the sentinel node 5 min after injection.

Static Imaging

The anterior view revealed at least four areas of focal uptake in the left groin. The first node that became evident during dynamic acquisition was considered to be the sentinel node. The overlying skin was marked.

Operative Findings

At operation, 1 ml of patent blue dye was injected subdermally. The site of the sentinel node was confirmed with the Neoprobe 1500. Through a 2.5-cm incision, the left groin was explored and the sentinel node was identified; it was hot and blue. There was another node proximal to this which was blue and less radioactive. Both nodes were biopsied.

Histology

Histology did not show any evidence of metastatic carcinoma in the sentinel nodes. Immunohistochemical examination of the lymph node was also negative.

Teaching Point

Penile carcinoma is one of the good indications for sentinel node biopsy. In this case, the status of the left groin nodes was determined with this technique in a patient who had lymphoedema of the right lower limb due to previous groin dissection.

Static Imaging

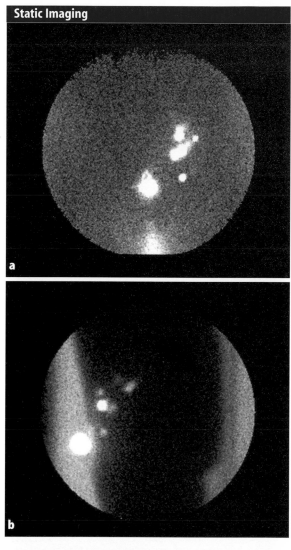

Anterior view **a**
Lateral view **b**

Histology

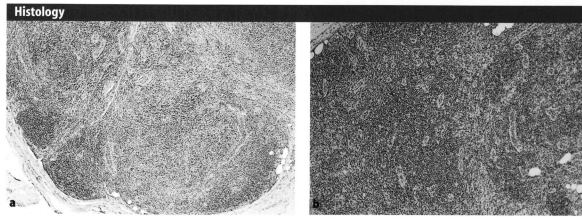

a Negative sentinel node (H & E)
b Negative sentinel node (MNF 116)

CHAPTER 12

Malignant Melanoma: European Practice *

Vivian Bongers, Inne H. M. Borel Rinkes,
Peter C. Barneveld, Marijke R. Canninga-van Dijk,
Peter P. van Rijk, Willem A. van Vloten

Introduction

For many years, the subject of elective lymph node dissection has been one of the most important controversies in the management of patients with malignant melanoma. The status of the regional lymph nodes is a critical component in staging patients with newly diagnosed melanoma, since lymph node involvement in these patients is known to be an unfavourable prognostic factor [1].

The majority (90%) of patients with primary cutaneous malignant melanoma present without clinically enlarged lymph nodes. However, it has been estimated that approximately 15% of these patients harbour occult lymph node micrometastases [2], and accurate diagnostic identification of such lymph node metastases in melanoma patients appears important. In an attempt to solve this problem, location of the first-echelon lymph node by means of the sentinel node procedure has gained increasing acceptance over the past decade. The sentinel node concept was introduced by Morton et al. [3], who initially used vital blue dyes to identify the sentinel node. However, this technique fails to localise the sentinel node in approximately 20% of cases, even in experienced hands. Subsequent reports have shown that the percentage of failures to identify the sentinel node is greatly reduced by using radiolabeled colloids in conjunction with a small hand-held gamma probe [4]. The presence or absence of metastases in the sentinel node has been demonstrated to accurately reflect the histology of the remainder of the nodal basin [5]. Additional dynamic lymphoscintigraphy is considered to be a more convenient alternative for lymph node mapping, particularly when separate lymph channels lead to nodes in separate lymph node basins. In such cases, omitting dynamic scintigraphy may result in incomplete nodal extraction, which could produce false-negative results [6, 7].

In the light of these results most centres have adopted a sentinel node methodology in which blue dye and lymphoscintigraphy are used in combination. However, since the accuracy of the blue dye technique is limited [3, 4, 8], we postulated that it might be sufficient to rely on lymphoscintigraphy alone if an optimal protocol is available. Therefore, the aim of this prospective study was to assess the accuracy of lymphoscintigraphy alone (without blue dye) for the identification of the sentinel node, using technetium-99m nanocolloid as the radiopharmaceutical, and two-phase dynamic/static lymphoscintigraphy. Concurrently, the incidence of alternative lymphatic drainage pathways as well as their impact on reliable nodal staging was assessed.

Since the sentinel node procedure is steadily gaining popularity for several tumour types [9–13], a uniform implementation of a standardised procedure would be advisable. In an attempt to evaluate the current practice, we sent a postal questionnaire to 136 nuclear physicians in 16 different countries in Europe. Based on the outcome of this first independent (non-commercial) survey, we report on the sentinel node procedure as practised on melanoma patients by 40 European nuclear medicine physicians from ten different countries and against this background present recommendations for routine implementation of the sentinel node procedure. The ultimate goal of the formulation of such guidelines is to attain uniformity and international exchangeability of results for optimal interpretation and quality assurance.

---

* First published in *Eur J Nucl Med* 26, 1999.

Materials and Methods

Between January 1995 and April 1998, 80 patients with a malignant melanoma, but otherwise in good clinical health, underwent lymphoscintigraphy for lymphatic mapping and sentinel node biopsy. None of them had palpable lymph nodes on clinical examination. All patients satisfied the following criteria. They had a histologically proven malignant melanoma, which had been excised with a small surgical margin. No skin grafting had been performed and the diagnostic excision had taken place less than 2 months prior to the sentinel node procedure. A wider excision of the primary site was performed simultaneously with the sentinel node procedure. Pregnancy was excluded. Detailed patient characteristics are listed in Table 1.

On the day of surgery an average amount of 80 MBq ^{99m}Tc-nanocolloid (Nycomed Amersham, plc) in 0.8 ml saline, divided in four equal portions, was injected intracutaneously on both sides of the scar of the diagnostic excision. Immediately after the ^{99m}Tc-nanocolloid injections, dynamic acquisition (20 frames of 60 s, 256×256 matrix) was started. Anterior and lateral static views were obtained after 1–2 h. The location of the sentinel node was checked with the hand-held gamma detector (TecProbe 2000, Stratec Electronic GmbH, Birkenfeld, Germany), and was marked on the skin with a cobalt-57 penmarker. Lymphoscintigraphy was performed with a single-head rectangular gamma camera (Elscint 609) equipped with a low-energy, high-resolution collimator. Images were obtained with a symmetrical 10% window over the 140-keV ^{99m}Tc energy peak. The gamma probe was used intra-operatively to again locate the sentinel node. This was done after wide re-excision of the primary lesion to minimise background radiation. Once the sentinel node has been excised, the lymphatic basin was checked for any remaining radioactivity and the radioactivity

Table 1.
Clinical variables and histopathological data of 80 patients with a malignant melanoma without palpable lymph nodes (Garbe et al., 1995 [26])

Characteristics	Number	Pos. SN [a]
Sex	35 male/45 female	
Age at diagnosis	46.7 years	
Age range at diagnosis	18–81 years	
Anatomic location [b]		
Back, thorax	29	5
Scalp, neck, upper arm	15	4
Lower trunk, leg, foot	30	3
Face, lower arm, hand	6	1
Breslow thickness		
<0.76 mm	1	
0.76–1.00 mm	4	
1.01–1.50 mm	26	3
1.51–3.00 mm	31	5
3.00–4.00 mm	8	1
>4.00 mm	10	4
Clark level		
II	4	
III	23	4
IV	49	8
V	4	1
Histologic subtype		
Superficial spreading melanoma	38	4
Nodular melanoma	22	5
Amelanotic melanoma	1	1
Lentigo malignant melanoma	1	
Malignant melanoma	18	3

[a] Pos. SN = tumour positive sentinel node.
[b] Classification into anatomical regions listed according to increasing risk of death.

of the sentinel node was confirmed. Histopathologic examination of the sentinel node was performed using routine haematoxylin and eosin staining techniques on serial sections. If this showed the sentinel node to be tumour positive, an elective regional lymph node dissection of the affected basin, including the site of the sentinel node biopsy, was subsequently performed.

In an attempt to assess the degree of variability of the methodology used throughout Europe, we sent a postal questionnaire to 136 nuclear physicians in 16 different countries in Europe, in May 1998. This questionnaire gathered the following information: (1) demographic data of the respondents; (2) the number of patients being investigated each year and the specific inclusion criteria (Table 2); (3) technical details of the sentinel node procedure (Table 3, 4) and (4) data about the surgical retrieval of the sentinel node by a gamma probe.

Results

Single Institution Evaluation of the Sentinel Node Procedure in 80 Patients

Lymphoscintigraphy with ^{99m}Tc-nanocolloid allowed sentinel lymphadenectomy in all draining node fields without any significant morbidity. In general, intra-operative tracing of the sentinel nodes was not problematic. Lymphatic transport of ^{99m}Tc-nanocolloid began immediately after administration of the radiopharmaceutical. A sentinel node could often be identified on the dynamic images within a few minutes. Lymph drainage patterns could be visualised in 79 of the 80 patients. Scintigraphy of one patient with a cutaneous malignant melanoma in the axilla failed to show a sentinel node owing to proximity of the injection site to the lymph node area basin. Despite adequate pre-operative visualisation, the sentinel node could not be retrieved during surgery in 2 of the 79 patients, in one case on account of a technical failure of the probe, and in one case when too few counts remained in the sentinel node 6 h after injection of the tracer. In all patients who showed multiple sentinel nodes at pre-operative examination, all of these nodes were accurately identified and excised during the operation. The sentinel

node contained metastases in 13 out of the 77 evaluable patients (17%). On subsequent selective regional lymph node dissection of the affected basin, only four of these patients (Breslow thickness 2.6, 5.5, 7 and 8 mm, respectively) displayed additional tumour positive nodes within the lymphadenectomy specimen (24%). One of these patients developed extensive haematogenous metastatic disease within 16 months postoperatively. In the other 11 patients the sentinel node was the only tumour containing node (Breslow thickness ranging from 1.1 to 4.2 mm). To date, none of the patients with a tumour-free sentinel node have developed regional or distant metastases during follow-up. The follow-up ranged from 2 to 42 months with a median of 21 months.

In 79 patients one to three sentinel nodes were visualised: one in 38 patients, two in 33 patients, and three in eight patients. Moreover, in 24 of the 41 patients with more than one sentinel node, multiple channels were seen to originate from the injection site – in 16 of them towards multiple sentinel nodes in only a single basin, in six patients towards two lymph node basins, and in two patients even towards three separate lymph node basins. In those patients with a malignant melanoma draining on multiple lymph node basins or on anatomically unpredictable lymph node basins, dynamic lymphoscintigraphy contributed significantly to the sentinel node procedure. Moreover, in 2 of the 13 cases with lymph node metastases, dynamic lymphoscintigraphy produced essential information. In one patient with a malignant melanoma of the scalp, dynamic lymphoscintigraphy showed two separate lymph channels to nonpalpable sentinel nodes on both sides of the neck, both of which proved to contain malignant disease (Fig. 2). In one other patient with a melanoma on

Table 2. Results of the European questionnaire about the sentinel node procedure in patients with a malignant melanoma. The number of sentinel node procedures in the different responding institutes is shown

No. of treated patients per year	No of institutes
< 12	8
12 – 24	12
25 – 49	7
50 – 99	9
> 100	4

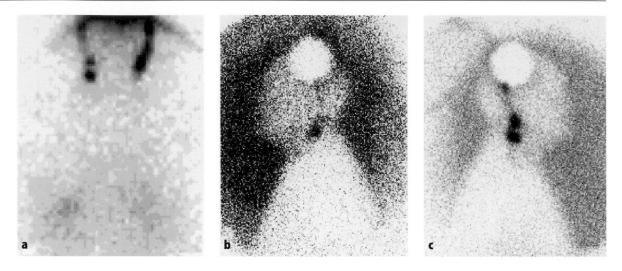

Fig. 1 a – c. Scans from an 81-year-old woman with a melanoma of the scalp. The early posterior dynamic phase of the lymphoscintigram (**a**) shows two dominant lymph channels to the right and left neck. The delayed scans (2 h after injection) in the left (**b**) and right (**c**) lateral position show the two sentinel nodes on both sides in the posterior triangle of the neck. Both of these nodes proved to be tumour positive

the left lower arm, lymph flow to both the left antecubital fossa and the left axilla was recorded. Each lymph channel met a single lymph node. The node in the antecubital fossa was found to be negative, while the axillary sentinel node was shown to contain tumour metastasis (Fig. 1).

Survey of the Practice of the Sentinel Node Procedure in Europe

Fig. 2. Scans from a 44-year-old woman with an amelanotic melanoma of the left lower arm. Early dynamic study recorded flow of lymph to the antecubital fossa (*arrow*), and to the axilla (*arrowhead*) where each met a single sentinel. The node in the axilla proved to be tumour positive, whereas the antecubital node was tumour negative

One hundred and thirty-six nuclear medicine physicians in 16 different countries received a questionnaire concerning the application of the sentinel node procedure in their institute. Two months later 83 replies from ten different countries

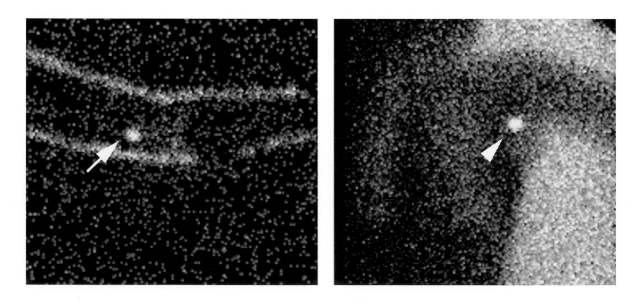

Fig. 3.
Range of Breslow tumour thickness as inclusion criterion for the sentinel node procedure in different institutes in Europe

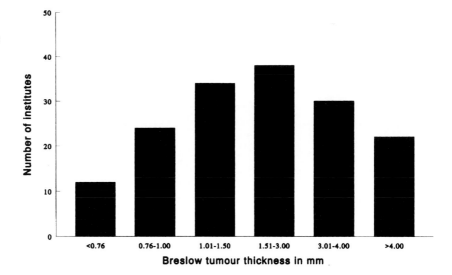

has been received, a response rate of 61%. Seventy replies had arrived after 1 month. At that time a reminding letter was sent to the non-responding institutes, whereafter the other 13 replies were obtained (16% additional response rate). Forty of the 83 responding nuclear medicine physicians were actively performing the sentinel node procedure (48%). The number of sentinel node procedures performed and the inclusion criteria of the different responding institutes are shown in Table 2 and Fig. 3. In 20 of the responding institutes the sentinel node procedure was only performed in patients with non-palpable lymph nodes, but in the other 20 institutes the procedure was performed both in patients with palpable lymph nodes and in those without. In 18 institutes the sentinel node procedure was always preceded by a diagnostic excision biopsy, in two institutes this was never done. In the other 20 responding institutes a preceding diagnostic excision biopsy was frequently the procedure of choice, but not always. The technical details of the sentinel node procedure are presented in Table 3, and the imaging data in Table 4. The discordance in the delivered dose of the radiopharmaceutical was striking: approximately half of the respondents used 40 MBq, while the other half administered 80 MBq. Also, the chosen interval between injection of the radiopharmaceutical and intra-operative retrieval of the sentinel node varied. Half of the respondents performed the operation on the sentinel node more than 12 h after the imaging procedure.

Thirty-six of the 40 respondents used a gamma probe for retrieval of the sentinel node during surgery. The other four used gamma camera imaging for sentinel node retrieval in combination with the blue dye procedure, but without using the gamma

Table 3. Results of the European questionnaire about the sentinel node procedure in patients with malignant melanoma: technical details

Technical details	No. of institutes
RPh	
^{99m}Tc-nanocolloid	32
^{99m}Tc-sulphur colloid	5
^{99m}Tc-Human serum albumin	3
Administration of the RPh	
Local, intracutaneously	40
Number of injections	
2	6
4	37
8	4
RPh dosage in MBq	
20 or < 20	8
40	14
60	5
80	13
Interval injection/surgery	
< 6 h	14
< 12 h	6
> 12 h	20
Use of the gamma probe	
Yes	36
No	4

RPh, Radiopharmaceutical.

Table 4. Results of the European questionnaire about the sentinel node procedure: imaging data

Imaging parameter	No. of institutes
Lymphoscintigraphy	
Only static	9
Two-phase	31
Camera collimator	
LE all purpose	20
LE high resolution	20
Matrix size	
64×64	5
128×128	28
256×256	13
Usage of a skin marker	
No	3
Ink	33
Cobalt-57	12

LE, Low energy.

probe. The majority used the probe with a collimator. The sentinel node was retrieved during operation by using both count and sound detection with the probe. In 26 of the responding institutes the nuclear medicine physician supported the surgeon during operation, in five other institutes this role was fulfilled by the nuclear technician, and in the other nine hospitals their was no support from the nuclear medicine department in theatre. If the sentinel node showed metastasis, a complete lymph node dissection was advised.

Discussion

Lymphoscintigraphy is based on the important observations of Morton et al. concerning the functional anatomy of regional lymph nodes [3]. More recently, the technique has been optimised by injecting a radioactive tracer as well as vital blue dye, and by using a gamma detector intra-operatively to facilitate localisation of the sentinel node [14, 15]. Subsequent studies have reported high reproducibility of this technique, depending on radiopharmaceutical, tumour and imaging parameters [16]. In the present study, using only ^{99m}Tc-nanocolloid as the tracer and the TecProbe 2000, surgical retrieval of the sentinel node was successful in 96% of cases. This success rate is comparable with those rates achieved using both the scintigraphy technique and the vital blue dye mapping

technique. Using blue dye alone, it is difficult to precisely localize the blue-stained nodes prior to skin incision, which may result in unnecessary dissection, and it is difficult to verify the removal of all sentinel nodes. Moreover, the blue dye causes staining of local tissue, and substantial experience is needed to achieve a high success rate [3, 4, 8]. In addition, adding blue dye to lymphoscintigraphy visualises the sentinel node in only approximately 60% of cases, while co-staining of other lymph nodes occurs. By using a small hand-held gamma probe, the lymph node is exactly located for a small incision in the overlying skin. However, vital blue dye could be of value in those cases with intra-operative obstacles (e.g. a primary tumour overlying the basin of interest), and/or technical problems (e.g. a marginal count rate in the sentinel node).

Lymphoscintigraphy, performed as a two-phase study of dynamic followed by static imaging, appears essential in identifying the physiological lymphatic flow through lymph channels to lymph nodes in individual cases. These images are valuable indicators of the drainage basin, (particularly in those cases in which the sentinel node is located outside usual nodal basins) and of sentinel node numbers. The phenomenon of melanomas draining to multiple basins has previously been described by several authors [7, 17–20]. In our study multiple draining basins were seen in patients with a primary melanoma on the trunk, the frontal scalp, the leg, the shoulder and the lower arm. Moreover, in 10% of the patients, the lymph drainage was located outside the expected nodal basins. These aberrant lymphatic pathways were mostly ascribed to the location of the primary, e.g. the midline of the back or the sternum, the so-called watershed areas. However, one patient with a malignant melanoma on the lower left side of the back showed a sentinel node in the left flank, and not, as expected, in the groin. The fact that functional imaging identifies lymphatic pathways and nodal bed drainage from the tumour site which would not have been predicted from classic anatomical approaches, has a direct bearing on surgical management and, therefore, on accurate regional staging. Failure to obtain dynamic images may lead to misdiagnosis of the sentinel node.

After more than two decades of debate, the sentinel node procedure may replace elective lymph node dissection in patients with a malignant melanoma, without clinically apparent lymph node spread, i.e. non-palpable lymph nodes [21]. Patients with a malignant melanoma of intermediate Breslow thickness (0.76–4.00 mm) have a high likelihood of occult regional lymphatic spread and should be selected for elective lymph node dissection. The rationale for this statement is grounded on data from prospective and retrospective studies which have suggested that patients with thin (< 0.76 mm) melanomas do well anyhow, whereas patients with thick (> 4 mm) melanomas have a high incidence of systemic tumour spread and, theoretically, may not be expected to benefit from local nodal resection [22, 23]. Therefore, in melanoma patients with a Breslow thickness > 4 mm the sentinel node procedure may still be of value as a research tool, but is not recommended as a standard diagnostic procedure for lymphatic staging. Besides, if any gain is to be obtained in this patient category, it will come from adjuvant systemic treatment, as is currently being investigated in the ongoing EORTC interferon trial. Concerning the clinical lymph node status, the sentinel node procedure is the procedure of choice in those patients with non-palpable lymph nodes.

In this article recommendations for standardisation of the sentinel node procedure have been formulated in order to ameliorate the generalisation of results. These recommendations have been based on the outcome of the first independent (non-commercial) survey of the clinical practice of the sentinel node procedure in patients with a malignant melanoma, and on our current experience. Since Breslow tumour thickness is the most significant prognostic factor for survival of patients with a localised melanoma and other pathologic and clinical parameters have not been conclusively verified as providing any additional information beyond that of tumour thickness [24], our inclusion and exclusion criteria for the sentinel node procedure are based only on tumour thickness and the clinical lymph node status. We recommend the sentinel node procedure for those patients with a melanoma, Breslow tumour thickness 0.76–4.00 mm and non-palpable lymph nodes. Recommendations for the sentinel node procedure are summarised in Table 5. Local, intradermal injection of 40 MBq ^{99m}Tc-nanocolloid in 0.8 ml, divided into four equal portions, around the diagnostic excision scar of the primary melanoma is followed by imaging, before the patient's scheduled surgery for definitive excision of the primary tumour with appropriate margins and excision of the sentinel node. Since we still use an older probe type with lower sensitivity, 80 MBq ^{99m}Tc-nanocolloid was used for adequate retrieval of the sentinel node, but with the introduction of the newer type probes, 40 MBq will sufficient for adequate retrieval of the sentinel node [25]. Two-phase lymphoscintigraphy appears essential for the reliable mapping of the sentinel node. Multiple projections may be required to image all drainage beds. If possible, the interval between injection and surgery should be kept between 6 and 12 h for optimal retrieval of the sentinel node by the gamma probe with a sufficient number of counts. Gamma camera imaging is limited to guide the surgeon to the sentinel node, because the lymphoscintigrams are static two-dimensional images. In addition, the skin projection of the identified sentinel node is based on gamma camera imaging and frequently lies several centimeters away from the actual radiolabelled node. Furthermore, the pa-

Table 5. Recommendations for the sentinel node procedure in malignant melanoma patients with a Breslow tumour thickness 0.76–4.00 mm and clinically negative lymph node status

1. Local, intradermal injection of 40 MBq ^{99m}Tc-nanocolloid in 0.8 ml, divided into 4 equal portions around the diagnostic excision scar of the primary melanoma.
2. Two-phase lymphoscintigraphy: dynamic imaging (20 frames of 60 s, 128 × 128 matrix, LEAP* collimator) followed by static images 1–2 h later (180 s per record).
3. For optimal retrieval of the sentinel node the interval between injection of the radiopharmaceutical and surgery should be kept between 6 and 12 h.
4. Intra-operative retrieval of the sentinel node with a gamma probe. Use of intradermal blue dye injections whenever difficulties in identifying the sentinel node are anticipated.
5. Histopathological examination of the sentinel node on serial sections.

* LEAP – Low Energy All Purpose.

tient's position on the operating table may differ considerably from that during lymphoscintigraphy. Therefore, the hand-held gamma probe, when used prior to incision, is useful for the exact localisation of the sentinel node, minimising the extent of the tissue dissection required. The gamma probe is placed on the marked skin surface over the sentinel node for 10 s to obtain a reading. After the incision the surgeon uses the probe, which has been placed in a sterile packing, to locate the sentinel node. Again, 10-s readings are obtained with the probe placed on the node, using sound and/or count reading. After excision of the sentinel node, count readings in the lymph node bed and then of the excised specimen are obtained. Excised lymph nodes are sent for histopathological examination on serial sections. Serial sectioning is considered essential in order to minimize false-negative outcome. The results of the questionnaire provided no indication as to the value of additional immunohistochemical staining. Also the literature offers no advice on the use of additional immuno-histochemical staining to judge lymph nodes in malignant melanoma patients. Recently, in our hospital, additional S100 and HMB45 staining of the serial lymph node sections has been introduced, but these results are preliminary and evaluation is still ongoing. The isolated use of ^{99m}Tc-nanocolloid for the sentinel node procedure has been verified as rational, but the additional use of blue dyes is very simple and can be very helpful, especially in those cases in which intra-operative difficulties (e.g. a primary melanoma very close to the anatomical lymph node basin) and/or technical problems (e.g. a low count rate) are anticipated. The presence of a nuclear medicine physician during the operation is recommended for optimal execution of this multidisciplinary approach.

Finally, assuming that the sentinel node procedure complies with the standard of care in patients with malignant melanoma as outlined in this article, how much growth in sentinel node procedures may be expected? A population-based study [24] has indicated that approximately 40% of patients who present with a primary malignant melanoma satisfy the criteria for the sentinel node – procedure. Extrapolating from the current Dutch situation with an approximate annual incidence of malignant melanoma of 1700 cases and 320 sen-

tinel node procedures per year, a 50% increase in sentinel node procedures is to be expected in the coming years.

In conclusion, the sentinel node concept is a rational approach for the selection of patients who could, theoretically, benefit from early lymph node dissection of the affected basin. This new strategy is now being applied in an increasing number of institutes. We consider the survey presented here as a first step towards a standardised sentinel node technique throughout Europe. This will lead to optimal exchangeability of data and, thus, to improved staging of patients with a malignant melanoma of intermediate thickness.

References

1. Balch CM, Soong SJ, Murad TM, Ingalls AL, Maddox WA. A multifactorial analysis of melanoma III. Prognostic factors in melanoma patients with lymph node metastasis (stage II). *Ann Surg* 1981; 193:377–388
2. Slingluff CL, Stidham KR, Ricci WM, Stanley WE, Seigler HF. Surgical management of regional lymph nodes in patients with melanoma. Experience with 4682 patients. *Ann Surg* 1994; 219:120–130
3. Morton DL, Wen DR, Wong JH, Economou JS, Cagle LA, Storm FK, Foshag LJ, Cochran AJ. Technical details of intraoperative lymphatic mapping for early stage melanoma. *Arch Surg* 1992; 127:392–399
4. Krag DN, Meijer SJ, Weaver DL, Loggie BW, Harlow SP, Tanabe KK, Laughlin EH, Alex JC. Minimal-access surgery for staging of malignant melanoma. *Arch Surg* 1995; 130:654–658
5. Reintgen D, Cruse CW, Wells K, Berman C, Fenske N, Glass F, Schroer K, Heller R, Ross M, Lyman G, Cox C, Rappaport D, Seigler HF, Balch C. The orderly progression of melanoma nodal metastases. *Ann Surg* 1994; 220:759–767
6. Pijpers R, Collet GJ, Meijer S, Hoekstra OS. The impact of dynamic lymphoscintigraphy and gamma probe guidance on sentinel node biopsy in melanoma. *Eur J Nucl Med* 1995; 22:1238–1241
7. Uren RF, Hofman-Giles RB, Shaw HM, Thompson JF, McCarthy WH. Lymphoscintigraphy in high risk melanoma of the trunk: predicting draining node groups, defining lymphatic channels and locating the sentinel node. *J Nucl Med* 1993; 34:1435–1440
8. Albertini JJ, Cruse CW, Rapaport D, Wells K, Ross M, DeConti R, Berman CG, Jared K, Messina J, Lyman G, Glass F, Fenske N, Reintgen DS. Intraoperative radiolymphoscintigraphy improves sentinel node identification for patients with melanoma. *Ann Surg* 1996; 223:217–224
9. Cascinelli N, Morabito A, Santinami M, MacKie RM, Belli F. Immediate or delayed dissection of regional nodes in patients with melanoma of the trunk: a randomised trial. *Lancet* 1998; 351:739–796
10. Krag D, Weaver D, Ashikaga T, Moffat F, Klimberg VS, Shriver C, Feldman S, Kusminsky R, Gadd M, Kuhn J,

Harlow S, Beitsch P. The sentinel node in breast cancer. A multicenter validation study. *N Engl J Med* 1998; 339: 941–946

11. Koch WM, Choti MA, Civelek AC, Eisele DW, Saunders JR. Gamma probe-directed biopsy of the sentinel node in oral squamous cell carcinoma. *Arch Otolaryngol Head and Neck Surg* 1998; 124:455–459

12. Senthil Kumar MP, Ananthakrishnan N, Preva V. Predicting regional lymph node metastasis in carcinoma of the penis: a comparison between fine-needle aspiration cytology, sentinel lymph node biopsy and medial inguinal lymph node biopsy. *Br J Urol* 1998; 81:453–457

13. Decesare SL, Fiorica JV, Roberts WS, Reintgen D, Arango H, Hoffman MS, Puleo C, Cavanagh D. A pilot study utilizing intraoperative lymphoscintigraphy for identification of the sentinel nodes in vulvar cancer. *Gynaecol Oncol* 1997; 66:425–428

14. Alex JC, Weaver DL, Fairbank JT, Rankin BS, Krag DN. Gamma probe-guided lymph node localization in malignant melanoma. *Surg Oncol* 1993; 2:303–308

15. Glass LF, Messina JL, Cruse W, Wells K, Rapaport D, Miliotes G, Berman C, Reintgen D, Fenske NA. The use of intraoperative radiolymphoscintigraphy for sentinel node biopsy in patients with malignant melanoma. *Dermatol Surg* 1996; 22:715–720

16. Kapteijn BAE, Nieweg OE, Valdés Olmos RA, Han Liem I, Baidjnath Panday RKL, Hoefnagel CA, Kroon BBR. Reproducibility of lymphoscintigraphy for lymphatic mapping in cutaneous melanoma. *J Nucl Med* 1996; 37: 972–975

17. Kapteijn BAE, Nieweg OE, Muller SH, Liem IH, Hoefnagel CA, Rutgers EJT, Kroon BBR. Validation of gamma-probe detection of the sentinel node in melanoma. *J Nucl Med* 1997; 38:362–366

18. Norman J, Cruse CW, Espinosa C, Cox C, Berman C, Clark R, Saba H, Wells K, Reintgen D. Redefinition of cutaneous lymphatic drainage with the use of lympho-scintigraphy for malignant melanoma. *Am J Surg* 1991; 162:432–437

19. Uren RF, Howman-Giles R, Thompson JF, Quinn MJ. Direct lymphatic drainage from the skin of the forearm to a supraclavicular node. *Clin Nucl Med* 1996; 21:387–389

20. Leong SPL, Steinmetz I, Habib FA, McMillan A, Gans JZ, Allen RE, Morita ET, El-Kadi M, Epstein HD, Kashani-Sabet M, Sagebiel RW. Optimal selective sentinel node dissection in primary malignant melanoma. *Arch Surg* 1997; 132:666–673

21. Reintgen D, Balch CM, Kirkwood J, Ross M. Recent advances in the care of the patient with malignant melanoma. *Ann Surg* 1997; 225:1–14

22. Sim FH, Taylor WF, Prithcard DJ, Soule EH. Lymphadenectomy in the management of stage I malignant melanoma: A prospective randomized study. *Mayo Clin Proc* 1986; 61:697–705

23. Veronesi U, Adamus J, Bandiera DC, Brennhovd IO, Caceres E, Cascinelli N, Claudio F, Ikonopisov RL, Javorski VV, Kirov S, Kulakowski A, Lacour J, Lejeune F, Mechl Z, Morabito A, Rode I, Sergeev S, van Slooten E, Szczygiel K, Trapeznikov NN, Wagner RI. Delayed regional lymph node dissection in stage I melanoma of the skin of the lower extremities. *Cancer* 1982; 49:2420–2430

24. Barnhill RL, Fine JA, Roush GC, Berwick M. Predicting five-year outcome for patients with cutaneous melanoma in a population-based study. *Cancer* 1996; 78: 425–432

25. Tiourina T, Arends B, Huysmans D, Rutten H, Lemaire B, Muller S. Evaluation of surgical gamma probes for radioguided sentinel node localisation. *Eur J Nucl Med* 1998; 25:1224–1231

26. Garbe C, Büttner P, Bertz G, Burg G, d'Hoedt B, Drepper H, Guggenmoos-Holzman I, Lechner W, Lippold A, Orfanos CE, Peters A, Rassner G, Stadler R, Stroebel W. Primary cutaneous melanoma. Prognostic classification of anatomic location. *Cancer* 1995; 75:2492–2498

CHAPTER 13

A Preliminary Study of Cost

Elliot Howard-Jones

Introduction

Breast cancer is the most common malignancy in women, accounting for 18% of all female cancers. Most patients who are diagnosed with breast cancer presently undergo surgery as an in-patient. This consists in wide local excision (WLE) of the tumour, and axillary lymph node dissection (ALND) in order to stage the disease. The patient will then stay in hospital for, typically, about 5 days, and will then be followed up as an out-patient.

This chapter explores the resource implications of an alternative treatment, whereby essentially the patient would still undergo WLE of the tumour but would also have a sentinel lymph node biopsy (SLNB), which would determine the status of the primary lymphatic drainage node. The status of the sentinel node would determine whether the patient would proceed to an ALND. From an economic point of view, this could generate savings over the present treatment, as the procedure without ALND should particularly reduce postoperative in-patient stay and complications. This chapter attempts to define the workings of a model that can be used in calculating this cost. Due to the extremely small sample sizes of the three groups, the findings can only be regarded as preliminary.

Resource Use in Breast Cancer Treatment

Patients will consume hospital resources when they receive either form of treatment. Therefore, for this particular study, five categories of resource use were defined. The first category is operating theatre usage. In any surgical treatment, the length of the operation will be a significant factor in the total level of resources consumed by the patient.

The second category of hospital resource use is the length of stay in hospital. Obviously, the more invasive the procedure, the longer the recovery time in hospital will be. There is also the risk of a higher level of complications with more invasive procedures, but this has been dealt with separately.

The third resource use is the identification of the sentinel node, involving both the use of the radiopharmaceutical and the time spent in Nuclear Medicine mapping the sentinel node. This relates only to those patients who have SLNB.

Fourthly, histopathology tests are undertaken on all patients who undergo breast surgery, but patients who have SLNB will have different tests to those who have the standard treatment.

Finally, an attempt has been made to cost the complications that arise from surgery, and to determine whether there is a different level of postoperative complications in patients who have ALND, and the level of cost associated with such a difference.

Throughout the model, both overheads and depreciation of capital equipment have been excluded, as their method of inclusion is to some extent subjective, and by focussing on costs, and not charges, it may also be easier to make comparisons with other centres.

The data from the UCLH trial relate to three sets of patients:

1. Patients who have undergone WLE and SLNB only, with no axillary clearance ($n = 7$)
2. Patients who have undergone WLE, SLNB and ALND ($n = 17$)
3. Patients who have had conventional treatment with WLE and ALND ($n = 30$)

The number of patients in each of the groups is small, and as such the data are used primarily for the purpose of illustration of the model. Often, one patient has severely affected the mean. As will be seen, some of the standard deviations prove that the spread of the data is very large, and this makes reliable estimates of the population mean difficult. In terms of using averages for length of stay and operating time to estimate the resource use these data are also of limited value, but this will improve as more patients are included in the study.

Differences in Resource Use

Operation Costs

The resources used in the operating theatre can be divided into two categories: staff time and consumables used. Using this principle, data were obtained from the UCLH theatres monitoring system, which details the time at which a patient is anaesthetised, the start time of the operation, time of entering and leaving recovery, and so on. Using this information it is possible to calculate the time spent at each stage, and the staff time associated with it.

It has been assumed that the same numbers of personnel attend at each stage, and a cost per hour was developed for each by using an average grade of each staff member, employing payroll data.

Three aspects of the time that the patient has been in theatre have been costed:

1. Anaesthetic time – time spent by the anaesthetist and nursing staff in the anaesthetic room
2. Operation time – cost of the surgeon's actual operating time
3. Time in recovery – cost of the recovery nurse

The results for the three groups of patients are shown in Table 1. As can be seen, the standard deviations are large. This makes the task of drawing conclusions from the data difficult. There is

also an anomaly that needs explaining. Whilst the operation time for WLE & ALND seems reasonable at 63 min, it would be expected that the WLE & SLNB operation would take less time. The fact that it takes over 10 min longer can only be due to the learning process of detecting the sentinel node. Clinical estimates of the time it takes to find a node would suggest that it should take about 15 min, and the overall time taken for this operation should therefore be nearer 50 min than 80 min. Some studies from the United States would suggest that, over time, the technique of the surgeon will improve [1], and some reduction of this time should therefore result. The time should also therefore fall for the group of patients who have WLE, SLNB & ALND.

Whatever the restrictions of the data, they can be readily converted into average mean cost by using proportions of the hourly rate, as shown in Fig. 1. As can be seen from Fig. 1 and Table 1, the majority of the time, and cost, is accounted for by the operating time. Although the recovery time varies noticeably, it makes up a tiny proportion of the total cost, as the staff costs are relatively low. From these data we can calculate three significant costs. Firstly, the cost of the SLNB can be derived by subtracting the cost for the WLE & ALND group from that for the group which underwent WLE, ALND & SLNB; this is £81. Secondly, the ALND cost can be derived by subtracting the cost for the group which underwent WLE & SLNB from that for the group which had WLE, ALND & SLNB; this is £45. Finally, if we subtract the cost for the WLE & ALND group from that for the group which had WLE & SLNB, then we derive the extra cost of doing the SLNB even when the ALND is not undertaken, and this is £37.

This result suggests that there is a substantial 47% rise in costs, over the conventional treatment when SLNB is performed. This, again, relates to the

Table 1. Anaesthetic time, operation time and recovery time for the three groups of patients

	WLE & SLNB ($n = 7$)		WLE, SLNB & ALND ($n = 17$)		WLE & ALND ($n = 30$)	
	Mean	1 Standard deviation	Mean	1 Standard deviation	Mean	1 Standard deviation
Anaesthethic time (min)	10	5.39	9	3.22	12	4.96
Operation time (min)	79	29.82	100	23.30	63	26.84
Recovery time (min)	69	16.69	63	17.60	57	15.82

Fig. 1.
Relative contributions of operation, recovery and anaesthetic costs to the overall theatre costs, according to patient group

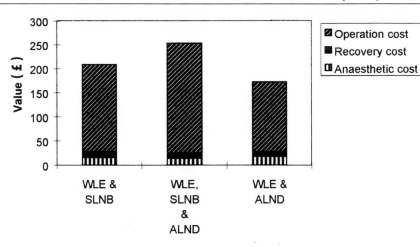

learning more of the surgeon performing SLNB. By comparison the ALND is relatively cheap, at only 12 % of the costs of conventional treatment.

The other result of note is that if the SLNB is performed per-operatively, and is found to be negative, avoiding an ALND, it will still be £ 37 more costly than the conventional treatment.

There are also other costs of operating that need quantifying. Firstly, there is the cost of the instruments that are used, in terms of their sterilisation (CSSD) cost. As the equipment used for each operation is the same regardless of the type, the cost for this was calculated at £ 104 per patient. The drugs and other consumables of theatres were assumed to vary with the length of the operation, and thus have been calculated by multiplying the hourly rate for these consumables, £ 86, by the length of time of operation. This breaks down for

the three groups of patients as shown in Fig. 2. There is relatively little variation between the three groups, and the pattern reflects that for the staff costs. The overall costs for each group (combining the costs detailed in Figs. 1 and 2) are therefore as shown in Fig. 3.

Length of Postoperative Hospital Stay

For all the importance of the operation costs, one must remember that the length of time that a patient stays in hospital costs up to 3 times the amount. The cost of the hospital stay has been calculated using an average daily rate, and multiplying by the length of stay of each patient. The daily rate included the cost of drugs, nursing time, dressings, linen and other miscellaneous expendi-

Fig. 2.
Cost of sterilisation (CSSD) and theatre consumables for the three groups of patients

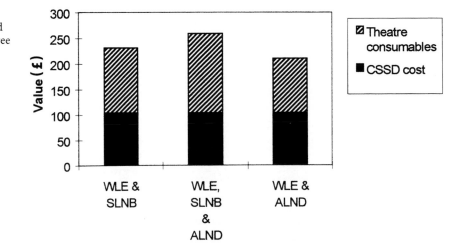

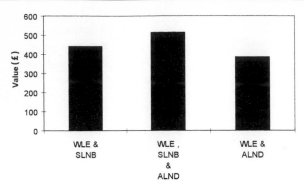

Fig. 3. Overall operation-related costs, according to patient group

Table 2. Mean duration of hospital stay (± 1 standard deviation) for the three patient groups

	Mean	1 Standard deviation
WLE & SLNB ($n = 7$)	3.43	1.49
WLE, ALND & SLNB ($n = 17$)	6.12	2.70
WLE & ALND ($n = 30$)	5.77	4.70

ture of the breast cancer ward. This revealed a cost of just under £ 103 per patient per day. The mean length of stay (and standard deviation) for each group is shown in Table 2. The findings are interesting. Whereas the groups which underwent axillary clearance, i.e. WLE, ALND & SLNB and WLE & ALND, had mean lengths of stay of 6.12 and 5.77 days respectively, with an associated cost of £ 627 and £ 591, the group WLE & SLNB (no axillary clearance) had a mean length of stay of just 3.43 days (£ 352). This translates into a saving of between £ 239 and £ 275, which is significant.

At this stage, it is worth noting again the small sample sizes of the three groups. Given these small sample sizes, it is not possible to estimate the population mean with any confidence, as some of the estimates would have a negative length of stay, which is clearly not possible. There does seem to be, however, a clear distinction between those patients who had ALND and those who did not.

Nuclear Medicine Cost

In order to locate the sentinel node, the patients are injected with a radiopharmaceutical the day before the operation and undergo mapping of the sentinel node. The injection of a blue dye just before operation helps to identify the sentinel node during the operation. As well as looking at the savings that might be made from the SLNB method of treatment, we must be careful to include costs such as these, which represent an area of increased expenditure for these patients. Obviously the expenditure above relates only to those patients who undergo SLNB, and is broken down into:

1. Hourly rate for the operator of the camera
2. Cost of the radiopharmaceutical

The cost of the operator is approximately £ 17 per hour, and a clinical judgment was taken to give an assumption that patients used, on average, about an hour of camera time in nuclear medicine. The cost of the radiopharmaceutical is £ 20 per patient. Thus, for each of the patients who have undergone SLNB a cost of £ 37 is incurred.

Histopathology

With conventional treatment, the nodes from the axillary clearance are sent for histopathology. Using the paraffin method, they are sectioned and stained, which costs about £ 20 per patient.

For the WLE & SLNB patient, just one node will have histopathology, but as frozen sections are taken, it is a more labour-intensive process, and so the cost is £ 16 per patient.

The main change as far as histopathology is concerned is the change to intra-operative testing, as this will be more significant than the change in costs outlined above.

Complications

There are significant advantages in moving away from ALND, as the detractors can point to the potential morbidity of arm oedema, nerve injury, increased risk of a frozen shoulder and additional recovery time. The removal of level III nodes carries up to a 37% risk of arm oedema [2]. However, to perform a total ALND is rare, and in partial ALND the risk of arm oedema is relatively low (2.7%–9.4%) [3]. In favour of SLNB, however, is the fact that as many as 70%–80% of patients with early breast cancer have pathologically non-involved lymph nodes, and would therefore not need ALND of any form.

This study has looked at the postoperative complications for all the patients, and the results for the three groups are shown below. The costing of the complications has followed exactly the same reasoning as above for operation time and hospital length of stay and, in addition, attendance as out-patients has been costed as £42, taking into account the cost of consumables and staff in the clinic.

WLE & SLNB

Of this group of seven patients, only one developed a complication (Table 3). The total cost of complications for the group was £42, which gives a mean of £6 per patient.

WLE, ALND & SLNB

Of the 17 patients in this group, five had complications (Table 4). The total cost of the complications for this group was £1526, with a mean of £90 per patient.

Table 3. Complications, and their cost, in patients in the WLE & SLNB group ($n = 7$)

Complication	Elements of cost	Actual cost (£)
Infection of wound	1 out-patient attendance	42

WLE & ALND

Of this group of 30 patients, five had complications (Table 5). The total cost for this group was £3343, with a mean of £111 per patient.

Conclusion

Table 6 shows a summary of the costs detailed in the preceding sections. In drawing conclusions from these data, two comparisons need to be made. The first comparison is the WLE & ALND group versus the group of patients who had WLE & SLNB only, and were thus spared the ALND and the associated longer length of hospital stay and higher complication costs. The second

Table 4. Complications, and their cost, in patients in the WLE, ALND & SLNB group ($n = 17$)

Complication	Elements of cost	Actual cost (£)
Axillary seroma	2 out-patient attendances	84
Some bleeding at breast site	1 out-patient attendance	42
Seroma at mastectomy site	1 out-patient attendance	42
Infected prosthesis	5 days LOS [a], 1 out-patient attendance, theatre time	637
Postoperative haemorrhage in axilla	6 days LOS, 1 out-patient attendance, theatre time	721

[a] LOS = Length of stay.

Table 5. Complications, and their cost, in patients in the WLE & ALND subgroup ($n = 30$)

Complication	Elements of cost	Actual cost (£)
Axillary wound	1 out-patient attendance	42
Axillary seroma	1 out-patient attendance	42
Wound infection at mastectomy site, debridement necessary	24 days LOS, 1 out-patient attendance, theatre time	2560
Postoperative haematoma in axilla	2 days LOS, 1 out-patient attendance	247
Breast wound cellulitic and axillary seroma	4 days LOS, 1 out-patient attendance	452

Table 6. Summary of cost (£) according to patient group

	WLE & SLNB ($n = 7$)	WLE, ALND & SLNB ($n = 17$)	WLE & ALND ($n = 30$)
Operation cost	440.51	513.06	383.29
Length of stay cost	351.55	627.28	591.29
Nuclear medicine cost	37.36	37.36	0
Histopathology cost	16.00	16.00	20.00
Complications cost	6.00	90.00	111.00
Total cost	851.42	1283.70	1105.58

comparison is the WLE & ALND versus the WLE, ALND & SLNB group to determine the extra costs of the sentinel node biopsy in patients who have to have an ALND after the sentinel node tests positive.

The first comparison, which is the saving resulting from not clearing the axillary basin, is £254 per patient. The second comparison, which concerns the additional cost relating to dissecting to axillary node after the sentinel biopsy, reveals that additional cost to be £198 per patient.

Before drawing conclusions from this, there is a further area of investigation that is needed which has not been costed in this chapter and is worthy of mention. This is the issue of the false-negative result of sentinel node biopsy. Potentially, the patient's disease will not be detected for some time after admission, and more costs may well be incurred than would have been the case if the node had been detected as positive and an axillary clearance performed. This has not been covered in this chapter, as a costing of this kind would need long-term data collection among patients who had not had ALND. This is outside the scope of the trial presently being undertaken.

Nevertheless, we can still draw conclusions using the costing results of this study, since it is possible to estimate the savings from the results of other trials. The literature would suggest that 70%–80% of lymph nodes in early breast cancer are negative. Taking a sample size of 100 patients, between 70 and 80 would have a saving of £254 each, which would generate to a total saving of between £17780 and £20320. The additional cost

of the 20 or 30 patients who would have to undergo axillary clearance, at £198, is between £3960 and £5940.

Taking the 70% lymph node-negative figure, the savings would total £17780 and the additional costs would be £5940; thus the net saving would be £11840 per 100 patients. With the 80% lymph node-negative figure, the savings would total £20320 and the additional costs would be £3960, yielding a net saving of £16760 per 100 patients.

The conventional cost of treatment on these patients would be £110558, and thus the sentinel node treatment would save between 11% and 15% of total costs. If the selection of patients for sentinel node biopsy could be improved then the number of patients who would need an axillary clearance as well should fall towards zero, and thus the savings of sentinel node biopsy treatment could rise to as high as 20% of total costs. These savings are meaningful, and will also result in a significantly better system of care for patients with early breast cancer.

References

1. Krag D, Weaver D et al. The sentinel node in breast cancer. *N Engl J Med* 1998; 14:941–946
2. Larson D, Weinstein M, Goldberg I et al. Edema of the arm as a function of the extent of axillary surgery in patients with stage I–II carcinoma of the breast treated with primary radiotherapy. *Int J Radiat Oncol Biol Phys* 1986; 12:1575–1582
3. Seigel BM, Mayzel KA, Love SM. Level I and II axillary dissection in the treatment of early stage breast cancer. An analysis of 259 consecutive patients. *Arch Surg* 1990; 125: 1144–1147

CHAPTER 14

The Future

Introduction

It is clear that significant developments will take place, on a wide front, in the fascinating field of sentinel node detection. At the very least this will lead to renewed interest in the study of the lymphatics in health and in disease. With the improved imaging techniques at our disposal and with better and more stable radiopharmaceuticals, the detailed study of patterns of lymph drainage and the mapping of lymph node basins will gain renewed focus. Much has been learned from the initial efforts of many and we now understand better the conditions which must be met in order to obtain reproducible and physiologically meaningful data. Further understanding the role of the lymphatic system in man will help to clarify the mechanisms and conditions which preside over the spread of disease and will also help to stratify patients more accurately into groups at high, low or intermediate risk. Developments are expected in most if not all of the areas covered in this text, and in this summary it will not be feasible to detail all the possible avenues of progress. Some are described below.

Radiation Detector Technology

Since radiation detectors are used widely in medicine, important groups within both academia and industry are dedicated to the development of new technology with improved imaging and detection characteristics. New radiation detector materials are being not just bench but also patient tested, and the past few years have been particularly exciting. New technology will develop on a broad basis, but it is to be expected that imaging and external detection will be combined and miniaturised such

that the new probes to be used in the operating theatre environment will combine the present probe merits of convenience and portability with the features associated with imaging. Work is in progress on imaging probes able to detect not just gamma rays (as for the technology described in this book) but also beta-emitting radionuclides, and both endoscopic and surgical probes have been developed. Another important area of progress is in the design of probes which minimise the effect of background radiation, which can hamper the successful identification of small volumes of tumour. Dual-energy imaging may also help in the detection of more superficial or deeper lying abnormalities. Sub-millimetre resolution has already been achieved, but the ultimate resolution will be imposed by the characteristics of the collimators used.

Optical Biopsy Probes

Elastic scattering spectroscopy is also under development as a means to obtain spectral imprints of tissue. An optical biopsy probe is under development – white light is passed through an optical fibre placed on the tissue under examination and the back-scattered elastic light is then analysed. Different tissues do exhibit different spectra. It would be possible to use this device in conjunction with sentinel node detection devices and obtain instant optical read-outs of the tissue characteristics of a number of sentinel nodes (Fig. 1).

Radiopharmaceuticals

At present all tracers used in the detection of the sentinel node demonstrate passive mecha-

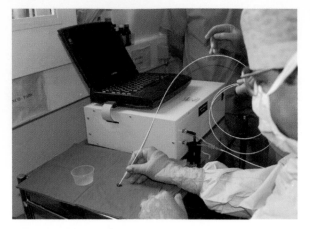

Fig. 1. Optical biopsy of the sentinel node

nisms of uptake which mainly reflect trapping and phagocytosis of labelled particles. In the next few years it will be necessary to have properly registered radiopharmaceuticals for the specific purpose of sentinel node detection. At present there are none. All of the relevant tracers in current use were developed years ago for the imaging of the reticuloendothelial system.

Significant batch to batch variations in particle size occur. This problem will be solved in the coming months. It is, however, uncertain whether the industry is prepared to develop an entirely new tracer for the sole purpose of sentinel node detection in view of the costs associated not just with the development process but also with the documentation/registration process now required by the various licensing authorities. Were it not for cost considerations, technology would be available for much improved tracers.

In the academic environment groups will continue to look at the development of tracers which take advantage of functional properties of the lymph nodes. Examples are tracers with specific receptor-associated uptake (Fc receptors or other small peptide-mediated lymph node uptake), some form of metabolic-mediated uptake (it is known that lymph nodes take up tracers such as labelled glucose) or antibody-mediated uptake (a number of possibilities have been and are being explored and described, often under the designation of radio-immunoguided detection/surgery).

Delivery of the Radiopharmaceutical

Interestingly technology is evolving here as well. A new approach to the delivery of tracer is the use of the J-Tip Needle Free Injector (National Medical Products Inc., USA). We have experimented with this device since it clearly presents a major advantage from the point of view of patient acceptance. If its use proves successful, reproducibility studies, which are still vital for improved understanding of the varying patterns of lymphatic flow, will be significantly facilitated, and the whole procedure will be rendered still less invasive.

The device which we have used is made of an almost standard syringe and plunger system, but at the proximal end of the device a small capsule of an expanding gas can be activated easily via a pressure point on the syringe outer layer such that the plunger is driven downwards by the rapid expansion of this gas. At high speed, the particles are delivered intradermally and with almost no pain to the patient. Studies are in progress to investigate the dispersion and the depth of delivery achieved with such devices, but interest is already extensive as judged by the achieved interaction with the pharmaceutical industry. An example of such a device is shown in Fig. 2.

Intra-operative Histological Diagnosis

At present, one of the limiting factors in the wider application of the sentinel node technique is the lack of a fast and reliable method of histological diagnosis. The false-negative rate of standard frozen section is unacceptably high, and this technique cannot be relied upon for routine intra-operative use. The technique of serial sectioning at 15 levels and standard immunohistochemical staining with cytokeratin markers, described by Veronesi et al. [1], has an acceptable accuracy but the significant increase in the operating time is a major drawback which renders its routine use impractical for most institutions.

The development of rapid immunostaining methods for frozen sections by Chilosi et al. is promising. Microwave irradiation is used to speed immunohistochemical analysis using "enhanced polymer one-step staining" (EPOS). The overall

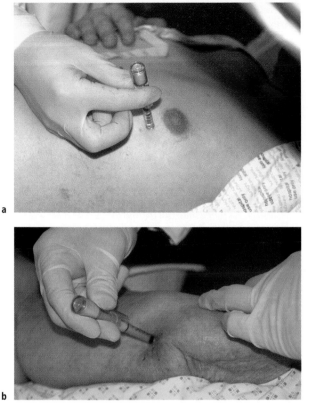

a

b

Fig. 2. J-Tip Needle Free Injector applied to **a** melanoma of the upper arm and **b** a male breast volunteer. (Provided by Mr. SGE Barker)

procedure takes less than 10 min and can be completed during surgery [2].

Intra-operative Imprint Cytology

Intra-operative imprint cytology is an area which requires more investigation. The preliminary data are very encouraging and we are presently evaluating the role of this method at our institution. The study performed by Fisher et al. [3] revealed that out of 50 patients who underwent axillary clearance, 21 had histologically confirmed metastatic disease; intra-operative imprint cytology detected 18/21 positive sentinel nodes. It was established that, had the technique of imprint cytology been used intra-operatively, 29 out of 50 patients may have avoided the operation, one would have had to have undergone extended axillary surgery and two would not have received further axillary surgery. The technical details and the pitfalls of this technique have been described in Chapter 10 of this book.

Clinical Applications

The utility of detection of the sentinel node in the management of patients with malignant melanoma is slowly becoming established, accompanied by the recognition that the technique represents a clear advance over past procedures. The jury is still out for patients with carcinoma of the breast, and data are only now beginning to accrue in other pathologies, such as colorectal and head and neck cancer. Only a few additional comments are pertinent at this stage.

An interesting area under investigation is the evaluation of breast cancer patients undergoing pre-operative neoadjuvant chemotherapy [1]. As the micrometastatic foci can be destroyed by chemotherapy, sentinel node biopsy can be performed prior to commencement of chemotherapy to appropriately stage the patient; if the sentinel node is negative, it may be possible to avoid axillary lymph node dissection, although the patient will need to be kept under close review for any recurrence in the axilla.

The implications which result from the detection of internal mammary nodes will need to be clarified. Marked variation in the detection of these nodes is reported by the different groups involved with this work, and at present there is no consensus on a management strategy for this group of patients.

As far as the sensitivity of the technique in breast cancer patients is concerned, have we already achieved an acceptable false-negative rate? Since the reported false-negative rate for the assumed gold standard management of axillary node dissection is of the order of 3% [4], it does seem that the minimum required target has nearly been achieved.

Clinical protocols will require rapid standardisation, but this will necessitate a major consensus conference.

There is a need for continuing education and training for this methodology to remain successful and reproducible. There is a definite learning curve associated with the technique, and a multidisciplinary team needs to be identified and supported.

There is a need for a cost-benefit study to investigate the implications of the technique in terms of resources and to assess its benefits and risks.

Only then will it be possible to provide patients with appropriate advice as to the relative merits of this new approach.

Issues regarding the quality of life and psycho-social well-being of patients will require careful consideration. In this era of minimally invasive surgery, patient acceptability of the procedure may well be high, but enthusiasm must be tempered by rigorous analysis of the risks and benefits. Patients will soon demand this procedure and clear explanations of its place in the surgical management of cancer.

The sentinel node concept has gained renewed importance and its impact on clinical management and surgical oncology can no longer be ignored. In the next few years, much new knowledge will be gained and the ultimate role of this methodology will be placed onto firmer ground.

The detailed and non-invasive investigation of the human lymphatic system will benefit us all, both patients and practitioners.

References

1. Veronesi U, Paganelli G, Galimberti V, Viale G, Zurrida ST, Bodeni N, Costa A, Chicco C, Geraghty JG, Luine A, Sacchini V, Veronesi P. Sentinel-node biopsy to avoid axillary dissection in breast cancer with clinically negative nodes. *Lancet* 1997; 349:1864–1867
2. Chilosi M, Lestani M, Pedron S, Montagna L, Benedetti A, Pizzolo G, Menestrina F. A rapid immunostaining method for frozen sections. *Biotech-Histochem* 1994; 69:235–239
3. Fisher CJ, Boyle S, Burke M, Price AB. Intraoperative assessment of nodal status in the selection of patients with breast cancer for axillary clearance. *Br J Surg* 1993; 80:457–458
4. McMasters KM, Giuliano AE, Ross MI et al. Sentinel-lymph-node biopsy for breast cancer – not yet the standard of care. *N Engl J Med* 339:990–995

Subject Index

#